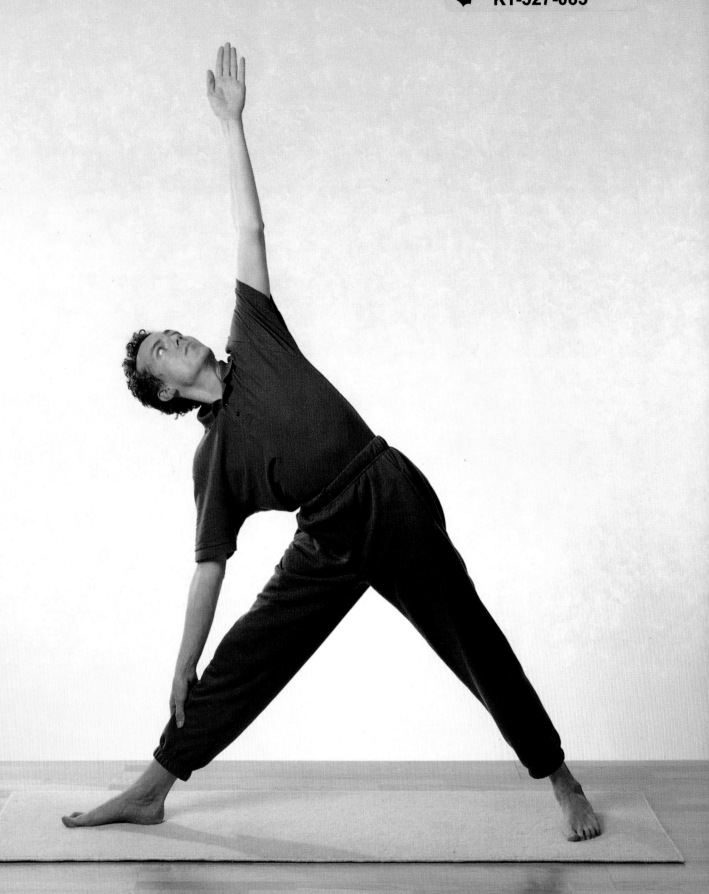

CONTENTS

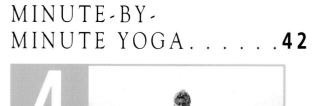

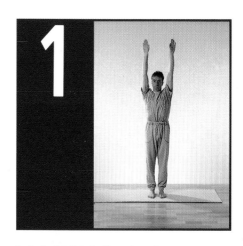

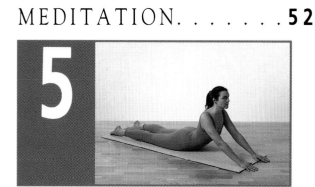

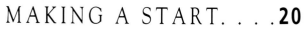

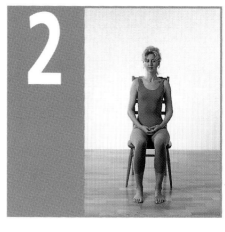

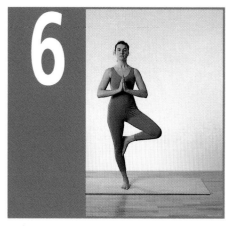

THE COMPLETE
YOGA
COURSE

Hazel Gilmour

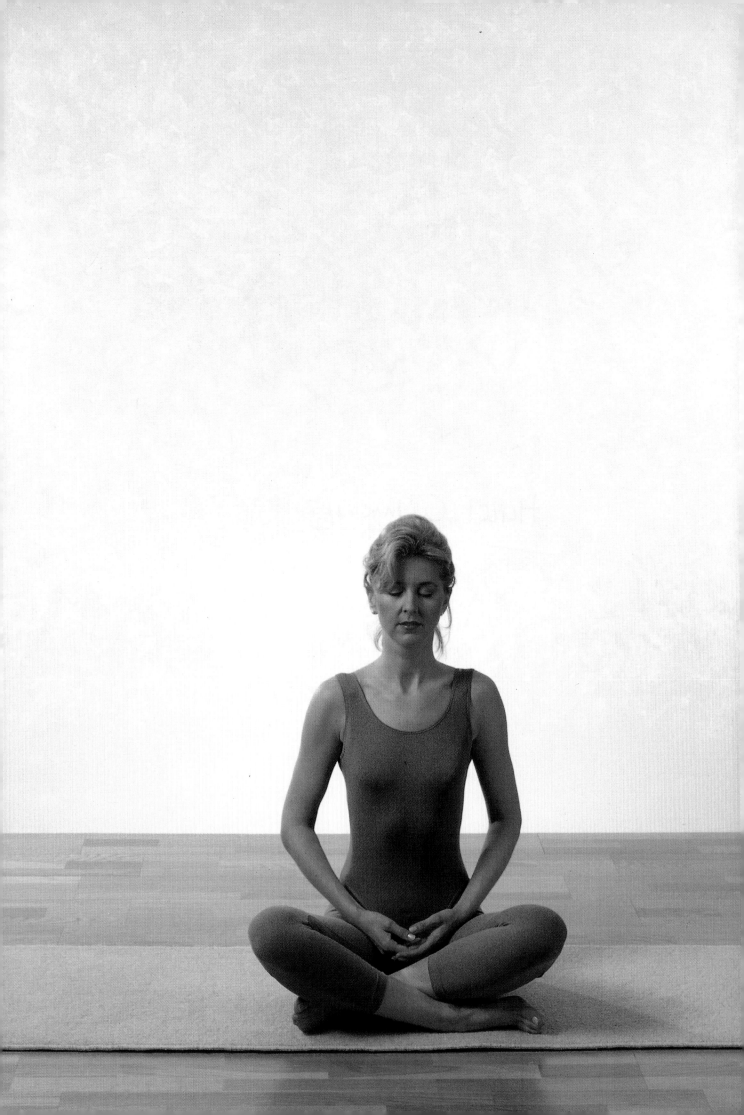

THE COMPLETE
YOGA
COURSE

HOWARD KENT

CHANCELLOR
PRESS

A QUANTUM BOOK

This edition published in 2000 by Chancellor Press
An imprint of Bounty Books, a division of
Octopus Publishing Group Ltd
2-4 Heron Quays
London
E14 4JP

ISBN 0-75370-365-3

QUMCYC

This book was produced by
Quantum Publishing
6 Blundell Street
London N7 9BH

Printed in Singapore by Star Standard Industries Pte Ltd

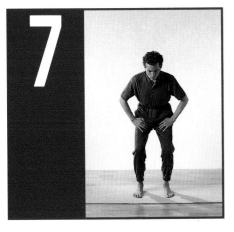

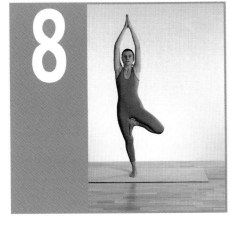

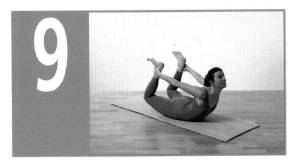

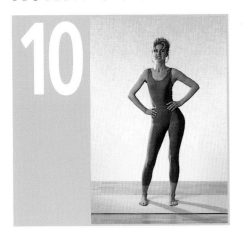

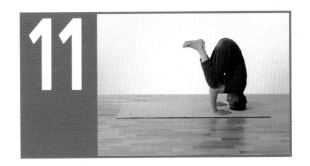

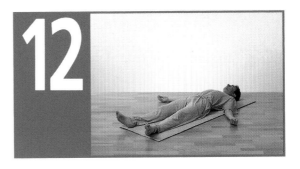

INTRODUCTION

To the question, why should an ancient Eastern concept attract millions of practitioners at the end of the twentieth century?, there is only one answer: because it works.

Yoga offers an attitude to life, from which a variety of practices have developed. First and foremost, yoga produces a feeling of peace, both in mind and body. In turn, this feeling stimulates both thoughts and actions, reminding us of the Latin tag: "Mens sana in corpore sano" ("A healthy mind in a healthy body").

The word "yoga" means unity or oneness – in other words, a feeling of being part of something. Yoga is one of the original concepts which today would be labelled as holistic. That means the body is related to the breath; both are related to the brain; in turn this links with the mind, which is a part of consciousness. The spelling of holistic, too, is a reminder that the word "whole" is derived from "holy" and therefore you cannot be a "whole" person unless you have a "whole" outlook on life itself.

It is not hard to realize that many of our ills today come from the feeling of isolation – *my* problems; *my* pains – a feeling that we are different and separated from others. In the last fifty years there has been a dramatic growth in the understanding of the universal problem now termed "unrelieved stress". At the core of such stress is the feeling of fighting a lone battle against great, often insuperable, odds. Today, thousands of doctors who know little or nothing about yoga nevertheless recommend patients to go to a yoga class to help them overcome a variety of stress-related problems. As more research is carried out, so the value of yoga becomes clearer and clearer.

Linking body and mind

Countless exercising plans are available today. New ones come into fashion and then fade away. Almost all of these depend exclusively upon working the body, quite unrelated to the conscious, thinking human being. It would be wrong to say such plans are useless, but their value is extremely limited, because they ignore the proven fact that the mind has a remarkable effect upon the body. Some people quite literally worry themselves to death; while others show a remarkable physical resilience simply because they remain calm and positive. As Buddha declared, some 2500 years ago, "You are what you think."

The aim of this book is to bring together, as simply as possible, the elements which make up life, so that, without making any undue demands, you can find body, breath, brain and mind working as one. It sounds difficult, but because it is a natural process, it is really quite simple once you understand what is happening.

The importance of being able to let go and relax in a world with increasing stress factors has become more and more obvious. Medical research, such as that undertaken in Britain by Dr Chandra Patel, showing the value of yoga techniques of relaxation in reversing long-held symptoms of high blood-pressure, has added a new dimension to the approach of yoga. In the last few years in America, Dr Dean Ornish has demonstrated that a yoga-orientated programme, involving a change in life style, can actually reverse symptoms of heart disease within twelve months. Through these and other important examples, it has become apparent that there is far more to yoga than performing a number of exercises slowly.

Achieving balance

The secret of yoga practice lies in a simple but important word: balance. It has always been stressed that yoga is not for one who eats too little, or for one who eats too much; nor for one who sleeps too little, or for one who sleeps too much. In every area, yoga represents balanced moderation. The idea seems easy enough, but following it through is not so simple in today's complex society. People tend to go at things either like a bull at a gate, or just to play around with them, expecting a great deal of benefit from very little effort. It is all to easy to say: "I don't want any of that philosophical nonsense; I'll just stick to the exercises." Unfortunately, the resulting benefit will be minimal and short-lived. Similarly, it can be just as deceptive to immerse oneself in the philosophy and create a state of mental indigestion!

This book enables you to take the middle path. By starting at the beginning and covering the ground slowly, it offers a programme that works for beginners and for relative newcomers. Many people who have attended classes – or are doing

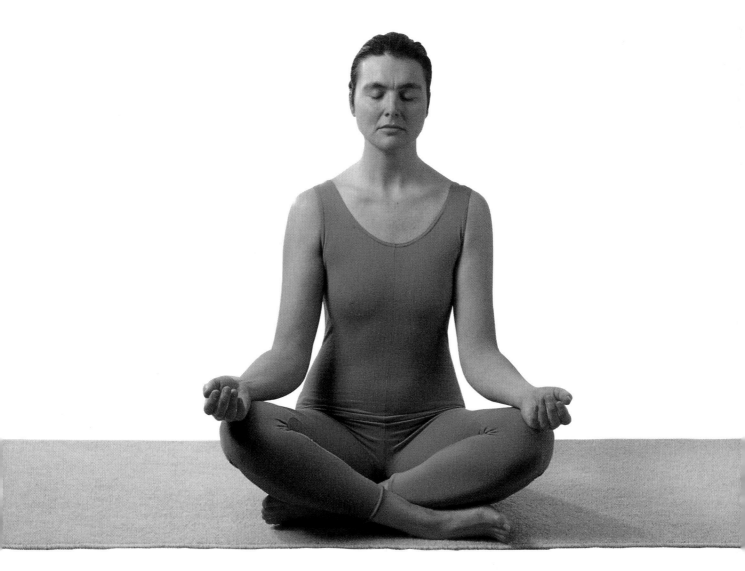

so currently – can benefit from having the main aspects of yoga outlined and developed in order. One aspect of taking a middle way is to be humble: in other words do not say, "I've done all that – I want to move on", but appreciate instead that it is important to retrace your steps and remind yourself of the basics. Life's lessons need to be learned thoroughly. You should remember, too, that the concept of the middle way applies to how you study, as well as to what you study. The role of the teacher is central, but this role implies not only how and what to instruct, but also how to encourage the student to develop personally both thought and practice.

Many thousands of people attend yoga classes each week, yet seldom, if ever, practise any aspect of the art on their own. Clearly this is unbalanced. The programmes offered in this book consist of a series of carefully thought-out suggestions. They do not oppose the teachings of a class leader, for there are many ways of approaching this vast subject. What is offered, instead, is a foundation upon which effective practice can be built.

Beware of fundamentalists in all walks of life, including yoga, because they can not appreciate the middle way.

The Purpose of Yoga

Buddha's statement – quoted earlier – "You are what you think," was made 2500 years ago. Around 300 years later, a great sage named Patanjali defined yoga as "controlling the activities of the mind".

The essence of yoga is to be in the driving seat of life. One of the great British scientists of this century, Sir Arthur Eddington, declared: "The stuff of the universe is *mind* stuff." In other words, real power lies in the mind – the very area that confuses and worries everyone so greatly.

Hatha Yoga

It is easy to make such statements, but much more difficult to put them into practice and, indeed, to live them. Over the centuries a number of interlinked yoga systems have been developed for this very purpose. The system

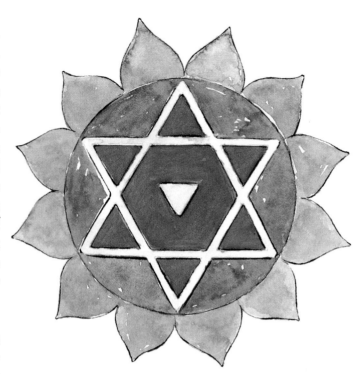

The Heart Centre

most used in the West is called *Hatha* (pronounced "hatta") *Yoga*. Virtually all general approaches come under this heading, although many people put names to their particular approach. Hatha Yoga involves the use of body positions, called *asanas*. (The word *Hatha* is a composite of *Ha* and *Tha*, which are symbols for sun and moon – the actual Sanscrit words are *Surya* for sun and *Chandra* for moon. These symbols signify positive and negative force in the electro-magnetic sense; thus *Hatha Yoga* is the yoga of polarized or balanced force.)

In addition to *asanas* the system includes a series of special breathing activities, known as *pranayama*. The translation of *pranayama* is "interruption of breath". In practical terms it involves a series of conscious controls of breathing which provide modifications of internal activities that in turn, stimulate, or sedate, brain activity as required for specific purposes.

Pranayama should not be confused with the enhancement of natural breathing or with the use of the breath in performing the *asanas*. While some *pranayama* techniques are outlined in this book, study of this subject is generally best carried out only under the guidance of an experienced teacher.

Hatha Yoga has a number of other practices not dealt with in this work. These can be studied later because confusion can easily set in if they are attempted too soon.

Hatha Yoga is an introductory system, leading us to greater things. The most celebrated text on *Hatha Yoga* is called the *"Hathapradipika"* (or "Compendium of Hatha Yoga") written in medieval times by a man called Svatmarama. He declared that he taught this *only* for the sake of *Raja Yoga*. The *Raja Yoga* system is specifically to bring about full control of the mind. A raja is the Indian equivalent of a king; thus *Raja Yoga* is called the King of Yogas.

Learning control

Control is a key aspect of yoga: control of the body, breath and mind. This may seem too much to try to undertake, but what is the alternative? It is to be out of control. This is hardly an attractive prospect and yet, if you stop to consider, the multitude of problems most people suffer from stem precisely from that absence of control.

The *asanas* of *Hatha Yoga*, for example, have a deep understanding of the principal areas of control of the body, including an understanding of the critical importance of the spine, which not only plays a major role in keeping

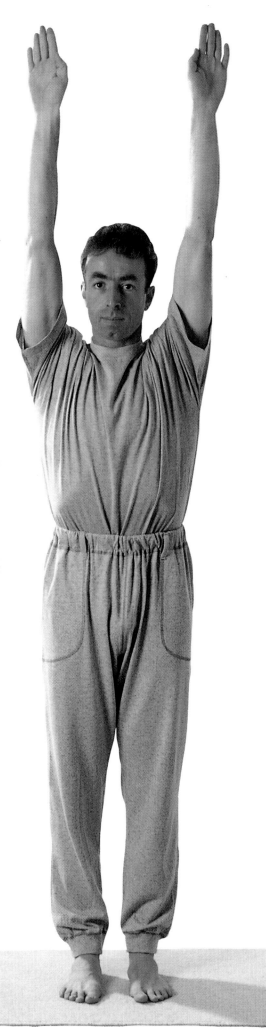

the body upright, but also provides the vital channel for the nervous system. Keeping the spine flexible, together with working the muscle groups of the trunk effectively, forms a central aspect of yoga postures. Controlled stretching – upwards, forwards, backwards, sideways – and twisting all play a major role.

The result is not simply a more supple and trouble-free back, but also an enhancement of digestive and abdominal organ function and, above all, a natural enhancement of effective breathing – the very core of life itself.

In turn, breathing affects outlook on life, for both oxygen and the body's electro-magnetic force are central to effective brain function. Thoughts, attitudes and emotions are all directly related to the state of body and breath. Agitated, depressed, unhappy thoughts damage breathing while, equally, poor breathing stimulates agitated, depressed, unhappy thoughts!

For almost everyone, life is a series of ups and downs, although we often feel there are far too many downs. You may look for steady happiness but, if you have any sense, you soon realize this is not the pattern of life. Balance, therefore, indicates a situation in which you can make the best of the ups, without trying to cling on to them, and accept the downs as quietly as you can.

Attitude of mind and control

To illustrate a valuable point, try this simple experiment with a friend.

Stand, holding one arm out to the side, clenching the fist to strengthen the muscles. Get the friend to stand behind you, placing one hand on the opposite shoulder to the outstretched arm and the other on the wrist of the outstretched arm. Now the friend firmly, but not jerkily, presses down on the wrist until the arm gives way.

Now put the arm out again and bring into your mind some problem you are currently concerned with, but are having difficulty coping with. Ask your friend to repeat the experiment. You will find that the arm is much weaker.

Put the arm out and once more bring the same problem back into your mind, but say to yourself this time that you know the problem can be resolved and you will not worry about it. The muscles are now much stronger than even at the first trial.

You can of course, try out the experiment on your friend in the same way. It could be argued that as you have been told what to expect, the result will be a subjective one, so why not try it out on someone without telling them what you believe will happen. You will find that the result is always the same.

Only one factor causes the change in this experiment: attitude of mind. As you have weak thoughts, the body also becomes weak. The brain has conveyed the weakness from mind to body.

Is yoga a religion?

One further aspect of yoga needs to be considered at this stage. Some people claim that yoga can be considered a religion or that it is simply a part of Hinduism, but what are the facts? Yoga, certainly, is not a religion. It has been described as, "The art of living, based on the science of living", which is an excellent description.

Thoughts of man's place in the universe, of the concept of God, and of the possibilities of heaven and hell have occupied humanity for countless years. Equally it became apparent that it was easy to *say* something, but far harder really to *feel* it and *live* it. Yoga arose as a series of controls and disciplines in which human beings could begin to experience the principles laid down in spiritual teachings and, by experiencing them, actually to live in accordance with them.

Although not a religion itself, yoga can enhance sincerely held religious beliefs. A number of excellent books have outlined the value

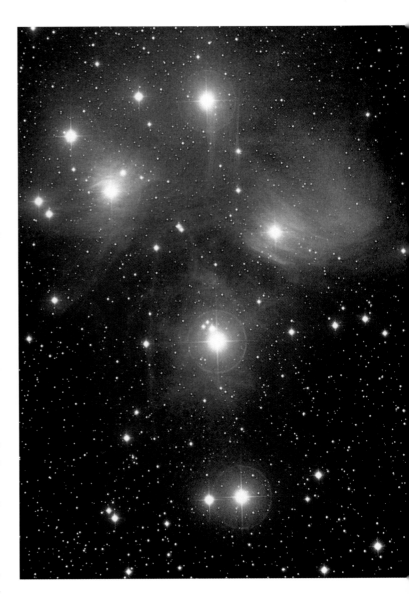

of yoga to Christians, for example. Religious fundamentalists, seeking to claim a monopoly of truth, often denounce yoga, but it is likely that a much greater number of people today would echo the words of Mahatma Gandhi: "Even as a tree has a single trunk, but many branches and leaves, so there is one true and perfect Religion, but it becomes many religions as it passes through the human medium. The one Religion is beyond all speech; imperfect men put it in such language as they can command and their words are interpreted by other men equally imperfect. Hence the necessity of tolerance, which does not mean indifference to one's faith, but a more intelligent and purer love for it. True knowledge of Religion breaks down the barriers between faith and faith."

Yoga, by enhancing true peace of mind, is an effective way of breaking down barriers, mental and physical.

HOW TO USE THE BOOK

There are few requirements for practising yoga. Clothing should not constrict the movement of the body. Light exercise outfits, such as those adopted for the martial arts, track suits and leotards are all suitable. There should be no constriction at the waist – no belts, for example. It is best to remove wristwatches and jewellery.

Most people like to have their own mat or thick blanket to practise on, but a well carpeted

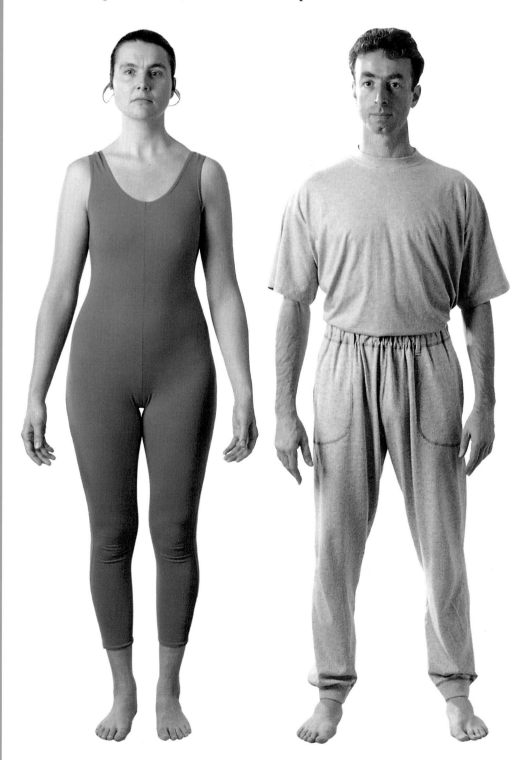

floor, free from dust, is quite suitable. It is important that your feet do not slip when you do standing poses. A wooden floor is ideal, but not essential. If you find your feet slipping on a carpeted surface, you may want to invest in a thin rubber mat (a camping mat would be fine).

Try to find a spot where you have sufficient room for all the movements. Adequate warmth is important. When relaxing you can cover yourself with a blanket, but avoid anything like a sleeping bag because it will constrict your body.

Naturally, you want peace and quiet. If it is practical, either take the telephone off the hook or switch on the answerphone. Teach yourself not to give into irritation if you are interrupted; such negative emotions can undo all the benefit you are working towards.

Regular practice

The word "discipline" has unpleasant connotations. Young children traditionally dislike the discipline of washing their necks, yet, if they are obliged to do so, it later not only becomes a habit, but they feel more comfortable and healthier as a result.

The regular practice of various aspects of yoga has the added advantage that the benefits quickly show themselves if the discipline is maintained. There are two most important aspects of the discipline, however. The first is that you must consciously give yourself to the practice, setting aside a period of time and concentrating fully. There is no benefit to be gained from merely going through the motions. In this busy world, people tend to do one thing while thinking or worrying about the next. In this way lie confusion, anxiety and ill-health. Ten minutes of complete concentrated yoga practice is far better for you than half-an-hour of unsettled thoughts. The second is that you must follow the programme best-suited to your own needs. It is possible to work to a book or a tape from time to time, but always remember each one of us has different needs. Becoming aware of these needs, and being able to deal with them, is central to yoga.

Yoga and Your Health

The aim of all yoga techniques is to get the best result using the minimum of energy. Because "making an effort" has become so much a part of our contemporary outlook, a number of cautions must be given to those taking up yoga practice.

• If you have any reason to believe you have a condition which affects your health, please seek advice before starting. Consult a qualified yoga teacher or your doctor.

• Those being treated for heart conditions or hypertension (high blood pressure) can benefit greatly from yoga, but should avoid inverted postures and take seriously the admonitions not to strain to achieve results.

• Forward bending should be avoided by those with a hiatus hernia.

• Asthma and bronchitis can be greatly improved through yoga. Asthmatics should slowly and gently learn to prolong the out-breath.

• Severe lung conditions will cause tissue damage. The stronger breathing techniques should be avoided, but quiet natural breathing should be practised regularly.

• If you find that any posture causes pain, withdraw slightly. Listen to your body and never strain it.

• Premenstrual tension is countered by yoga, but a woman teacher should be consulted for specific advice.

• There are books available on yoga and pregnancy (see Bibliography). There are no general rules as constitutions vary greatly. Again, consultation is the best course.

Millions of people all over the world now practise yoga regularly. Over the past 20 years, the Yoga for Health Foundation has not heard of anyone practising in their own home who has in any way damaged his or her own health as a result. On the contrary, countless letters have attested to the benefits which have resulted.

DEVELOPING A PROGRAMME

Today, people are invited to follow all sorts of different exercise programmes. If any one of these contained "the truth", all the others would fade away; many, however, contain elements of truth that have to be adapted to personal requirements.

The poet Kahlil Gibran encapsulated the proper outlook for yoga when he wrote:
"Say not, 'I have found the truth,' but rather, 'I have found a truth.'
Say not, 'I have found the path of the soul.'
Say rather, 'I have met the soul walking upon my path.'
For the soul walks upon all paths."

In this book, suggestions for building up a regular programme of practice are offered at the end of months two to eleven. But these are suggestions only, designed to stimulate study and personal decisions. Some postures, such as the Rabbit, are described but do not appear on the "Continuing the Programme" pages. This does not mean that they should not form a part of regular practice, but how they may fit in is

a matter for personal decision. To build a programme for yourself, take the following factors into consideration:
So far as the physical aspect of postures is concerned, relate to your own body and its needs but do not necessarily regard a disinclination to practise something you find difficult as a message from the body. It is more likely the consequence of a lazy attitude.

Bear in mind the principle of balance, which is at the core of yoga. The need for mental balance can affect which postures you choose to perform; the need for physical balance should determine the order in which they are performed. Many postures are always followed by a counter-posture. For instance, a stretch forward should be followed by a stretch backwards.

"Aims for the month" provides a focus for that particular month. Bear that in mind as you learn the new activities for that month.

"Thought panels" complement the activities, providing guidance and stimulating awareness of the interaction between body and mind.

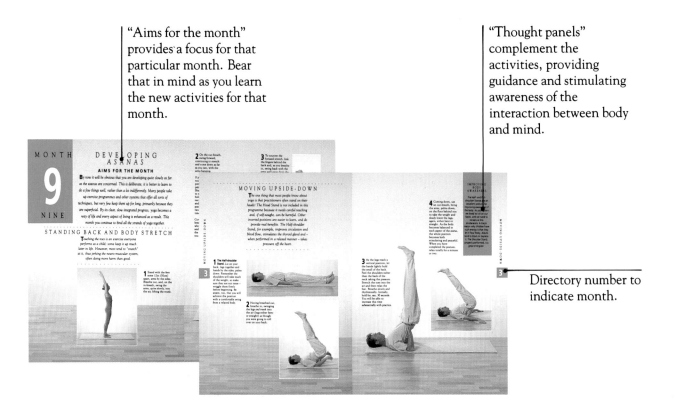

Directory number to indicate month.

Introduction to each month's programme. It is important to read this before you start developing your daily programme for each month. Remember that these programme spreads offer a series of examples: the final decision is yours.

Each strand of your yoga practice — postures, breathing, visualization, relaxation and meditation — has been given a different colour.

The pictures act as an aide-memoire. Refer back to the relevant pages if you need to study the posture or to refresh your memory.

Arrows lead you through the programme.

Some postures are paired together, either because you are comparing one with another, or because certain postures are always followed by certain counter-postures.

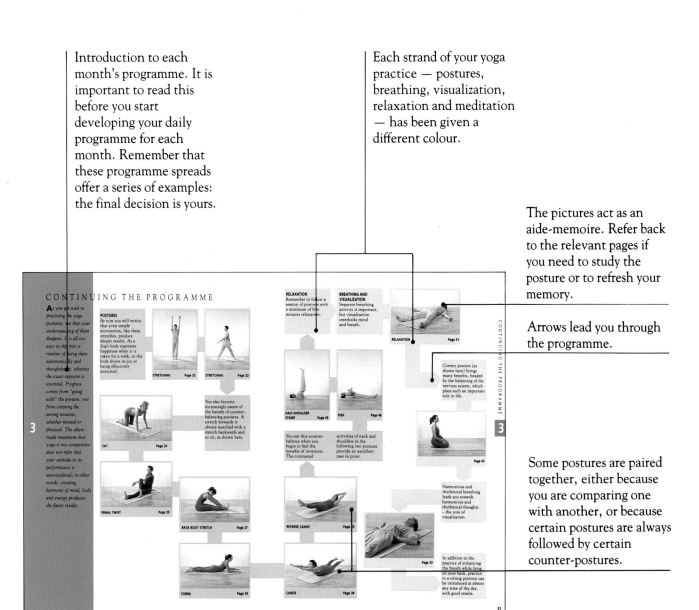

Remember that postures, relaxation, visualization and meditation are all integral aspects of life. Do not try to mix them up into a salad, but ensure each plays its rightful role.

As you develop a daily programme, constantly refer back – right to the beginning. You cannot remind yourself too often of the principles, and the different aspects of practice. Approach the whole business sensibly and happiness, health, peace and a sense of fulfilment can be yours.

Starting Off

If you can, set aside a specific time each day for practice. Allow at least one and a half hours to digest a small snack or two hours for a meal before you begin. This applies to all postures, including breathing, visualization and meditation. It is important to allow digestion to proceed unhampered.

The length of your practice will depend on the time you have available and the postures you choose to include in your session. However, it is better to do ten minutes than to skip practice altogether.

It makes sense to practise each new posture until you can remember the steps without needing to refer constantly to the instructions. It is wise to reread the instructions from time to time to ensure that you are doing the posture correctly and have not left out steps.

Some people may feel comfortable doing the same sequence each day, others will prefer variety. In any case, right from the start, develop the habit of looking through the portion of the book you have studied, remind yourself of the points made and make your own choice of what you plan to do.

MAKING A START

AIMS FOR THE MONTH

Slow progression is essential in yoga. Never forget that the central aim is to control the mind and this demands a quiet, methodical approach. Bear this in mind as you tackle the asanas (poses), even though you may feel you can already achieve more than is shown. Content yourself with working within limitations and achieving precise results. If you follow this principle, you will be doing only a small number of things by the end of the month, but you will be doing them well.

FREEING NECK AND SHOULDERS

The first areas of the body to stiffen up are the neck and shoulders. The muscles respond quickly to tension and poor posture, so simple movements to ease these areas should be performed during the day.

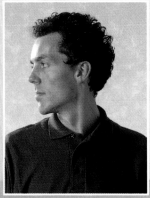

1 Sit, looking forwards. Breathe in then breathe out, turning the head to the right. Stop when the breath stops. Breathe in again without moving and again turn to the right on the out-breath.

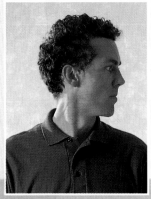

2 Hold the position and each time you breathe out feel the muscles relax. Breathing in, turn the head to the front and then, on the out-breath, turn to the left, following the same process as in step 1. Let several slow out-breaths relax the muscles.

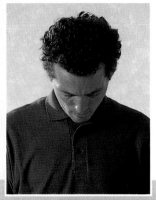

3 Bring the head to the front again on an in-breath and then, breathing out, drop the chin on the chest. Continue breathing rhythmically and each time you breathe out let the head drop further, with the chin pressing more into the chest.

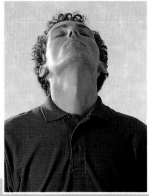

4 Breathing in, raise the head and then, breathing out, let it drop backwards. Clench the jaw. Continue breathing quietly and every time you breathe out allow the head to drop back a little further, stretching the front of the neck. Finally, breathing out, straighten the head.

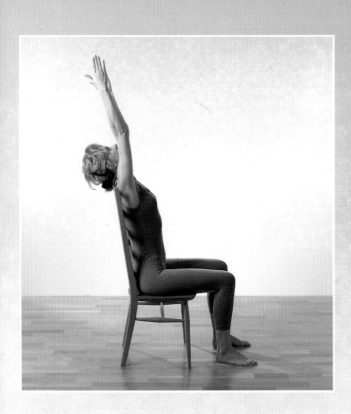

5 By combining the breath with a sweeping movement energy can be pumped quickly into the body. This is an excellent way to get you going when you are feeling stiff or lethargic, especially first thing in the morning. Practise it sitting on the side of the bed or in a chair, or sitting on the floor on your heels. Having breathed out, swing the arms sharply up over the head, breathing in deeply through the nose.

1

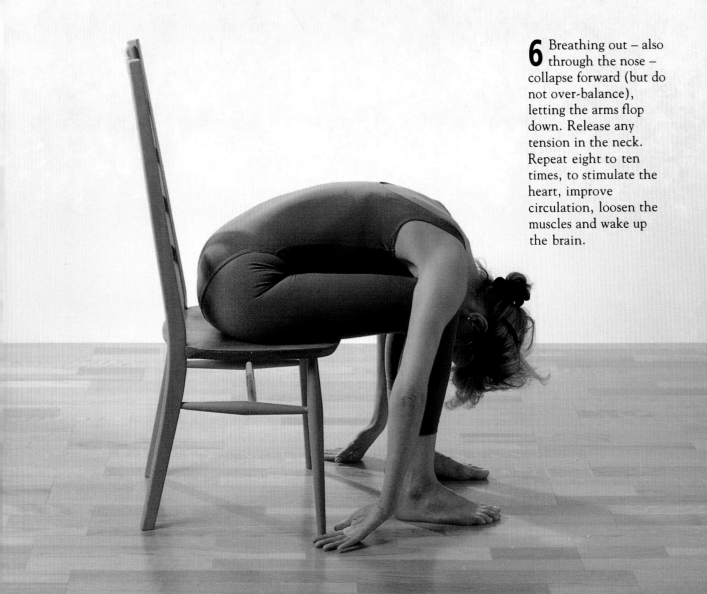

6 Breathing out – also through the nose – collapse forward (but do not over-balance), letting the arms flop down. Release any tension in the neck. Repeat eight to ten times, to stimulate the heart, improve circulation, loosen the muscles and wake up the brain.

STRETCHING

Stretching is important both for health and well-being. It should be carried out quite smoothly and slowly, not jerkily. This routine will tone the nerves and muscles, and improve circulation.

1 Stand erect, feet a few inches apart, palms of hands together, touching the chest. Hold the pose quietly for a minute.

2 Keeping the palms together, bring the hands on the head, with the elbows out. Take a deep, slow out-breath.

3 Breathing in, slowly stretch the arms upwards, palms together. Repeat steps 2 and 3 five times, breathing in on the stretch.

4 Next time you stretch up, open the palms forwards and raise the arms as high as possible.

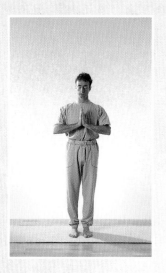 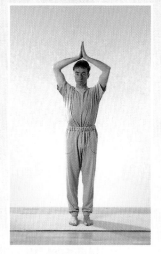 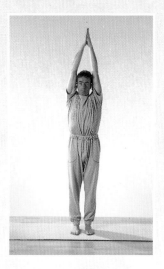 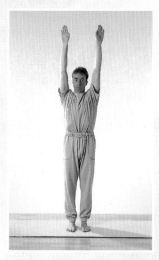

5 Then, breathing out, stretch forward, keeping the back as straight as possible.

6 Breathing in, straighten up and swing back, bending the knees to maintain balance.

7 Straightening up, breathe in and stretch to the right on the out-breath, with the arms straight. Repeat the same movement to the left, before once more stretching up as in step 4.

8 Finish by bringing palms together again, back down on to the head, then on to the chest and finally to the sides. Then let the head, shoulders, trunk and arms move freely as you swing from side to side.

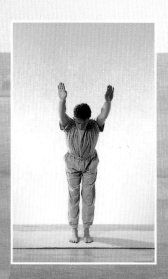 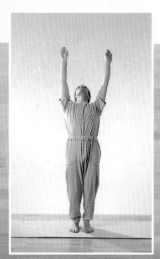 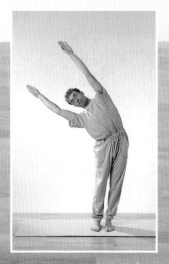 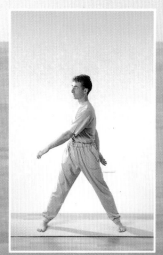

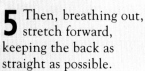

THE BREATH OF LIFE

Breath is life, but we also have great
voluntary control over our breathing. The key
to our energy system is in the diaphragm: a
strong sheet of muscle, attached to the bottom
ribs, separating the chest from the abdomen.
The diaphragm acts as a piston, literally
pumping the body's energy.

THE CONTROL OF BREATHING

Breath not only activates the body, it is the basis also of the functioning of brain and mind. Although it is an automatic function, controlling the breath can enhance daily life.

Worry, anger, agitation and excitement all affect the way you breathe, interfering with the harmony and the flow of energy. Paying sensible attention to the way you breathe is the foundation of effective living.

1

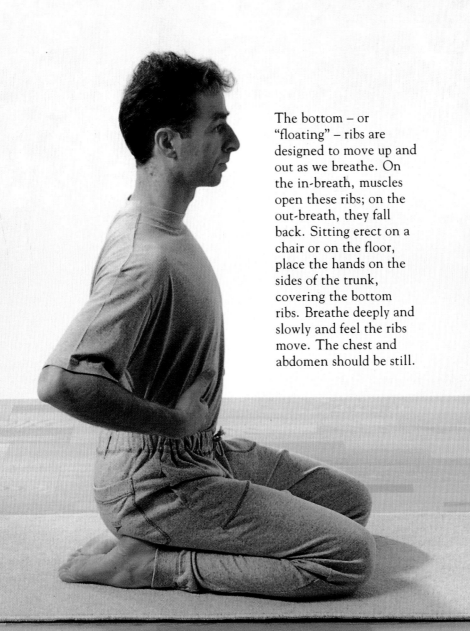

The bottom – or "floating" – ribs are designed to move up and out as we breathe. On the in-breath, muscles open these ribs; on the out-breath, they fall back. Sitting erect on a chair or on the floor, place the hands on the sides of the trunk, covering the bottom ribs. Breathe deeply and slowly and feel the ribs move. The chest and abdomen should be still.

THE SUPPLE SPINE

In the anatomy of human beings the spine is tremendously important. It provides essential flexibility and support, and it also provides a vital channel for the nerves, while its alignment affects the functioning of important muscles. We allow it to stiffen, or become distorted, at our peril.

When performing yoga movements for the spine, always remember that the body functions as a whole.

1 **The Cat.** Drop on to all fours, knees a little apart, palms facing forwards under the shoulder blades. Breathe in, dropping the back and raising the head. Hold for some seconds.

2 Breathing out, arch the back as high as it will go, dropping the head between the arms. Again, hold the position for some seconds. Repeat between 10 and 20 times.

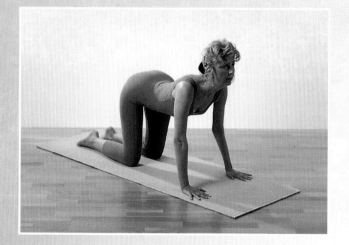

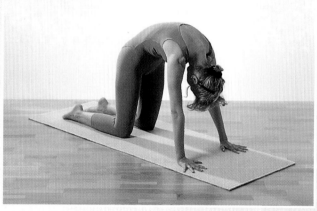

3 Finally, sink back on the heels, hands by the feet, palms facing upward, forehead touching the ground. Remain relaxed for two or three minutes. Get up quietly and slowly.

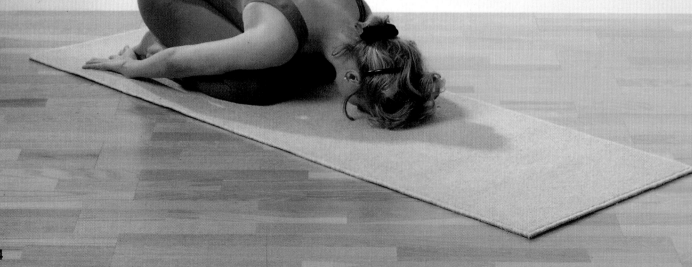

SPINAL TWIST

Twisting the spine can produce agonizing problems if adequate suppleness has not been maintained. Many people have turned sharply only to spend a long time in a medical corset.

This is a simple, but effective, version of the Spinal Twist. Remember that by moving slowly and then holding the position the elasticity of the muscles is enhanced. Sudden, jerky movements are always harmful. Really work the shoulder-blades: they will almost always twist round more than you think they can.

CONSIDERING THE WHOLE BODY

While the parts of the body need to be exercised, you must always consider the whole. Working on the spine is working on the entire being. The Cat is a slow dynamic movement; the Spinal Twist a static one. Each has its own special benefits.

When performing the Cat, let the mind dwell on sinuosity. With the Spinal Twist, clear the mind and let the maximum sense of relaxation follow.

1 Sit with your legs out in front of you, feet together, toes pointing upwards. Remember to sit upright, lifting the trunk a little, but not stiffly.

2 Bring the right hand to the back, feel where the spine is and bring the palm down on the floor, level with it, a few inches away from the back.

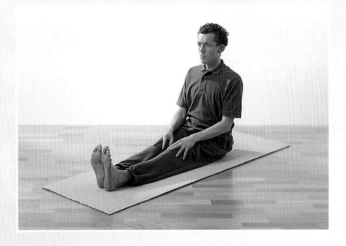

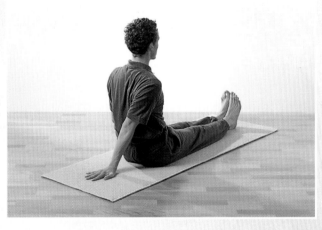

3 Bend the right leg, bringing it over the left leg at the knee-joint. Then bring the left arm against the right knee. Breathe in.

4 As you breathe out, swing the shoulders firmly but not sharply, to the right. Close your eyes and hold, breathing rhythmically, for at least 30 seconds. Repeat steps 1–4 on the other side.

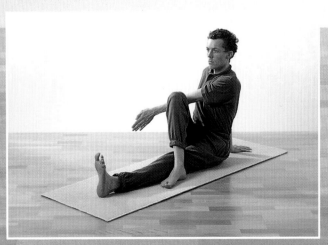

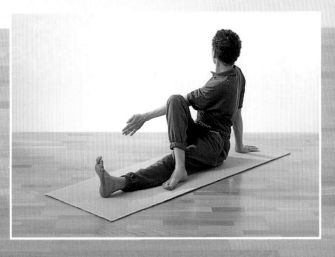

THE BACK BODY STRETCH

Back here refers to the whole posterior part
of the body. You have to remember that you
are constantly subject to the force of gravity.
Over the years this can compress the body and
needs to be countered by effective stretching.

The Back Body Stretch works from the
fingers to the toes: stretching the back of the
body and compressing the front of the trunk.
The majority of people allow the back to
become stiff. The more the mind dwells on
stiffness, the greater the problem becomes. Do
not regard the pose either as difficult or easy;
just say to yourself, "I am doing it", – and
follow the instructions carefully.

1 Sit on the floor with
the legs out in front,
feet a few inches apart,
toes pointing upwards.
Let the hands rest on the
floor, palms down by the
sides. Breathe slowly out
and then, as you inhale,
stretch the arms right up
in the air, lifting the
trunk. This will stretch
the spine and the
back muscles.

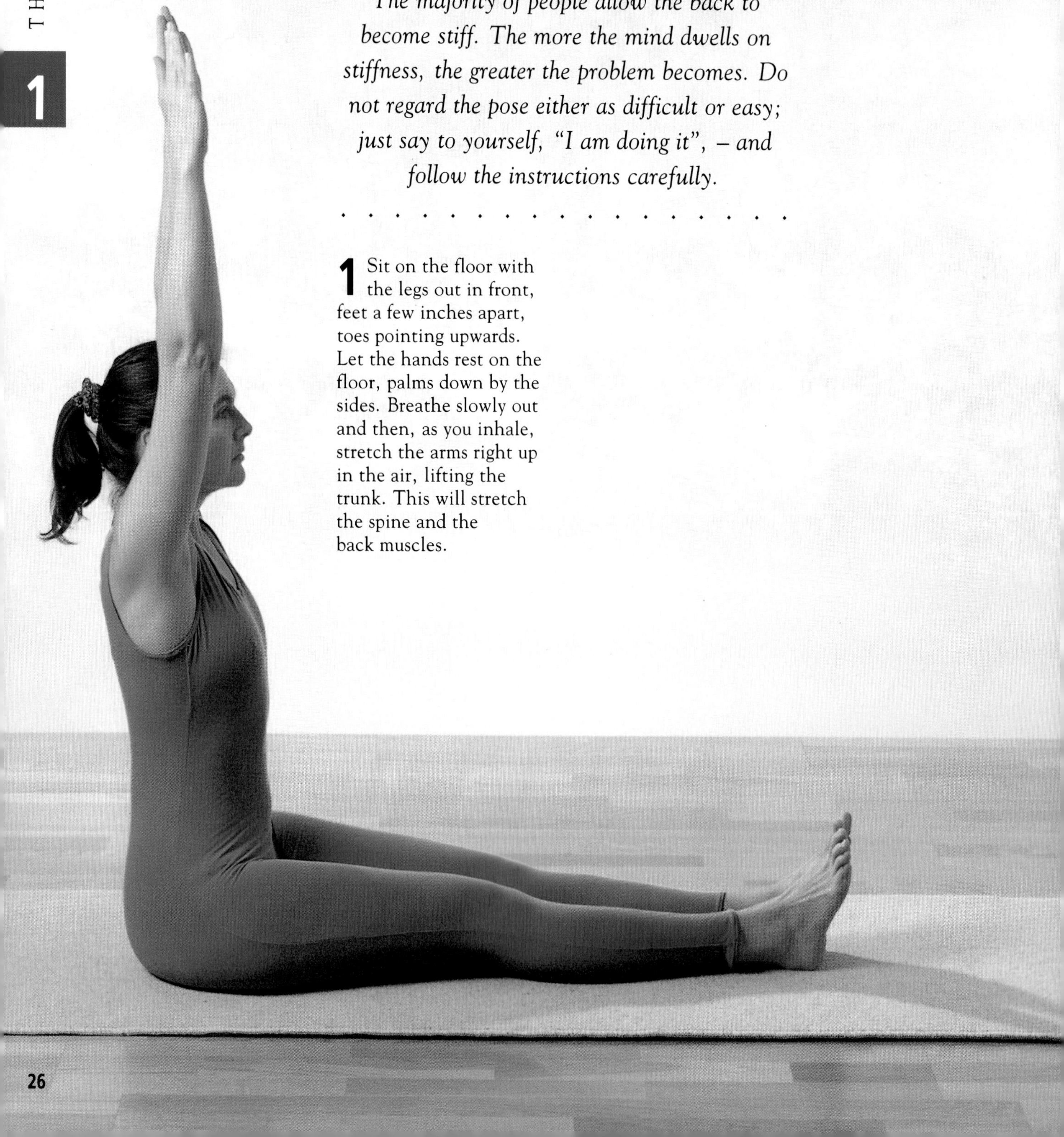

1

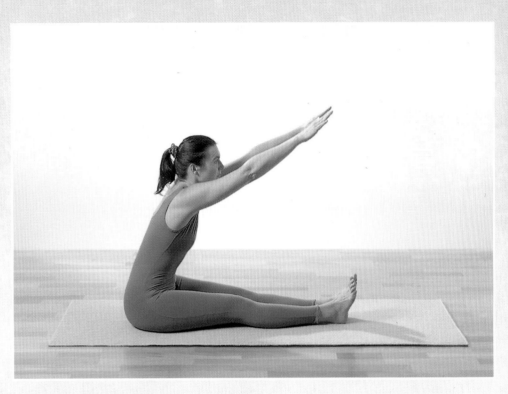

REMOVING STIFFNESS

This is a position which many people find difficult, but if you concentrate on the difficulty you will never progress. In most cases lower-back stiffness comes from lack of use and the muscles are perfectly capable of stretching. The same applies to the hamstrings. Right from the start, perform this *asana* quietly and slowly, and do not let considerations of time affect you.

1

2 As you breathe out, stretch slowly forward, maintaining the extended back, keeping the arms straight and the back of the legs on the floor. Breath and movement should come together exactly and the only thought should be one of reaching forward.

3 As the out-breath ends, let the hands hold the furthest part they can reach: the toes, the feet, the ankles or even the calves. Maintain a relaxed stretch with head hanging down. Hold, breathing gently, for at least 30 seconds. Come back up, stretching and breathing in. Then lie and relax.

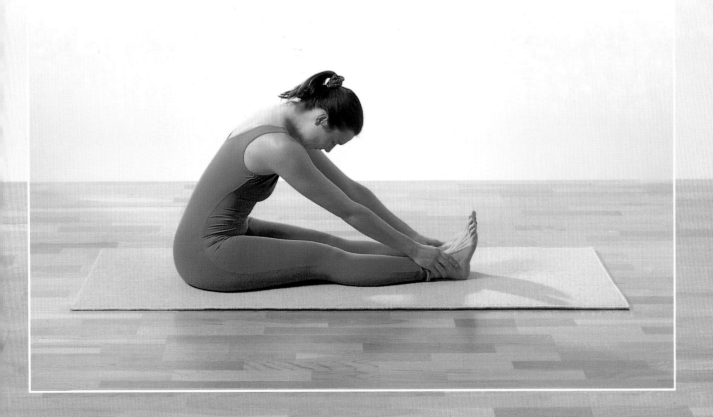

THE COBRA

Postures in yoga are balanced. Follow the
Back Body Stretch with the Cobra, so that
stretching and compression are complemented.
The Cobra mimics the snake rearing up,
which gives the clue to its performance.
It should seem a natural and inevitable
movement, in no sense should it be straining
for effect. In this way the front of the body is
stretched; both chest and abdomen are opened
up; the back and spine are compressed.
A good way to start is to think of it as a slow,
opening out dance movement, rather like the
petals of a flower unfolding.

1 Begin by lying on the
front, forehead on
the floor, arms by the
sides, palms upwards.
Feel comfortable
and relaxed. Breathe
out slowly.

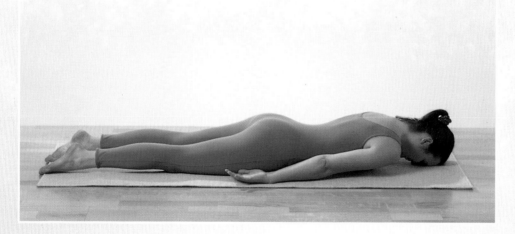

2 As you breathe in,
raise up the head,
neck, shoulders and
chest. As you feel the
need for extra support,
bring the arms in front,
palms down, to assist
the upward movement.

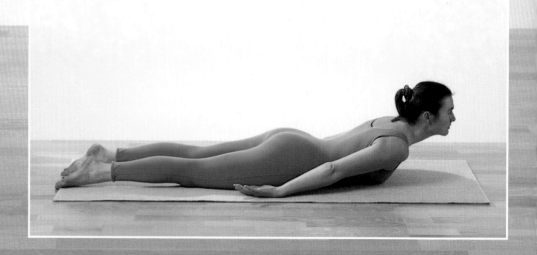

3 If your back is weak, or there is some muscular or spinal weakness, you can complete the position initially with the forearms resting on the floor. In many cases, however, this will be an interim position. As strength and confidence increase, transfer the pressure to the palms.

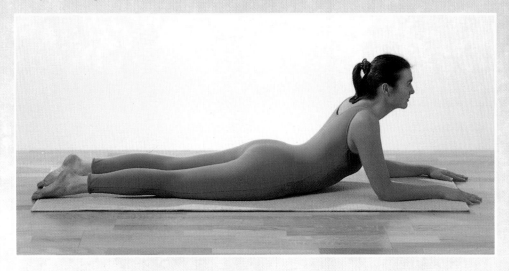

THE RIGHT ATTITUDE

Try to keep to the spirit of the posture. For example, people often tend to collapse out of the Cobra, but a snake would come down carefully and completely. This control is important, for it helps to establish our overall control. So when performing the Cobra, *be* the Cobra.

4 Continue to lift the upper body up, with the arms straight (not bent at the elbow). Adjust the hands to find the most comfortable position. Keep the hips and legs on the floor, so that the arms and trunk balance the upper body. Close the eyes and breathe slowly and quietly. Hold the pose for at least 30 seconds and come down on an out-breath, reversing the movement and then relaxing.

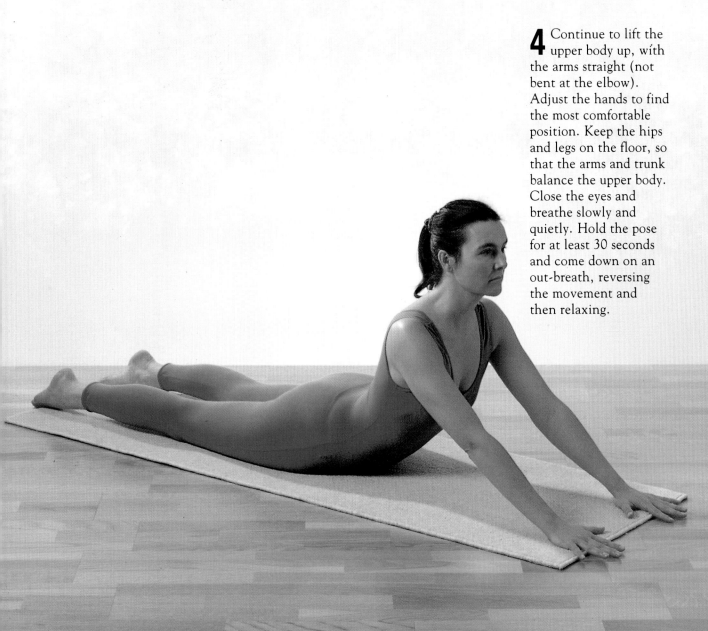

THE ART OF RELAXATION

*It is said that relaxation involves the most
difficult asana in yoga. It is called the Corpse
Pose, because it mimics how the body lies
after rigor mortis is over, when all tension
leaves the body. A better name, perhaps is the
Life Pose, because it is wholly open, displaying
neither agression nor fear. Remember
that relaxation is the opposite of activation.
Therefore, you cannot try to relax. In the
right conditions it will occur spontaneously.*

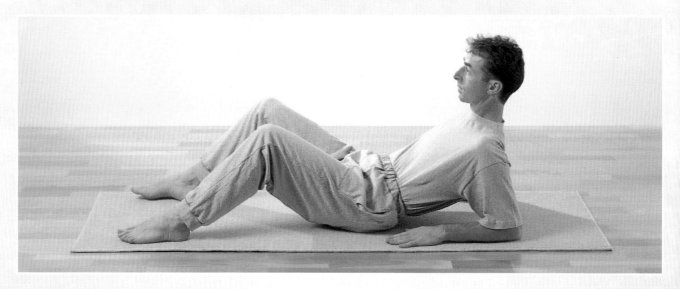

1 Come down
backwards on to the
floor with the knees
bent, resting on the
elbows, palms down.

2 Bring the back down
as flat against the
floor as possible, then
slide the legs down, with
the feet well apart.

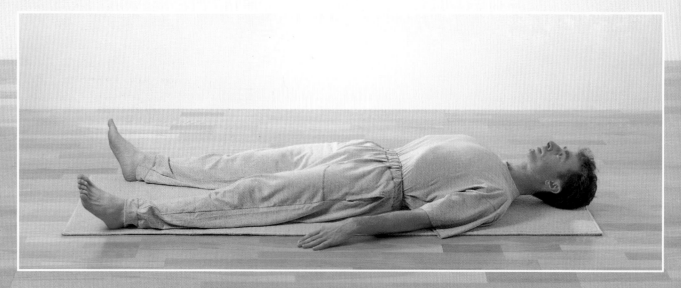

Relaxation is a process of observation without intervention. First of all observe the breath, which is quite automatic. Say to yourself, "I am not breathing; my body is breathing." Note that the tummy gently rises on the in-breath and falls on the out-breath. Feel the muscles relaxing and that the mind becomes more peaceful as they do so.

You cannot lead a balanced life without periods of relaxation. This is not the same as sleep, which is a combination of restfulness and specific internal activity. Relaxation is the vital process of letting-go. While relaxation techniques can effectively be practised throughout the week, remember the body and mind relax best after some form of physical activity.

· · · · · · · · · · · · · · · · ·

TIMING OF RELAXATION

Every yoga session ends with a period of relaxation. Practising at home, initially a five-minute period will be as much as you can achieve. Gradually increase, up to 15 to 20 minutes.

Brief periods of similar relaxation should also be interspersed through any session of *asanas*. The balance between being active and being able to let go is an extremely important one, as tension, unduly retained, is very damaging.

3 Move the arms away from the trunk, and roll the palms outwards. Let the mind consider the various parts of the body, looking for areas of tension. When practising relaxation, avoid concerning yourself with time. Initially, the mind is likely to do the opposite, telling you to be up and doing! Don't worry about this; let the process develop slowly but surely. Keep the eyes gently closed and do not lose awareness of the quiet breathing pattern.

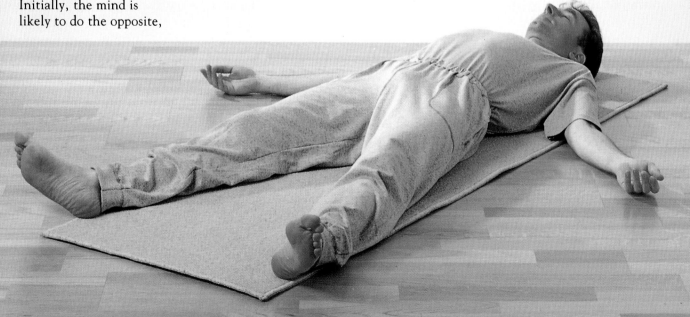

WIDENING THE SCOPE

AIMS FOR THE MONTH

During the first month you began to remove tension from the body, learned the vital role of the breath and started to relax. In the second month, comes a deepening understanding of respiration and of the power of the mind. You learn to increase the range of movements a little and to start to translate this into a daily programme. As you do so, you develop a greater degree of control over how you breathe – and from this you start to see that you can exercise this control over life itself.

· ·

ENHANCING THE BREATH

The bottom ribs play a decisive role in breathing (see page 23). Bad posture and agitated thoughts damage the breathing process, but with controlled breathing, the mind and body can be restored.

· · · · · · · · · · · · · · · · · · · ·

Sit or stand with the trunk upright. Do not slouch or throw the chest out. Become aware of your breath for a minute or two. Then begin to slow it down a little and ensure that it is rhythmical. Place the fingers lightly on the bottom ribs and become aware of their movement. The higher ribs play only a minor role and the abdomen is still. Concentrate quietly on the breath and its rhythmical movement. Be content to continue in this way for two or three minutes.

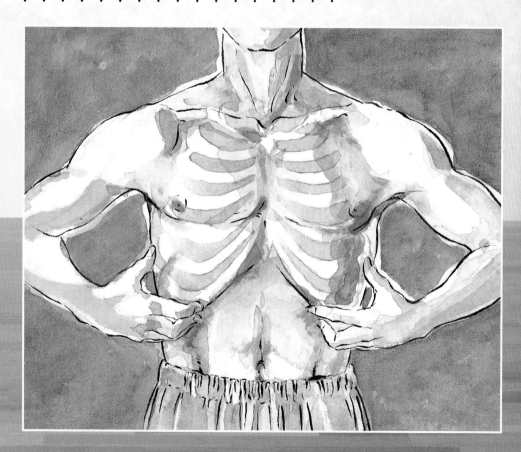

The diaphragm, attached to the bottom ribs, is dome-like and when you breathe in the movement of the ribs stretches and semi-straightens it. This helps the lungs to fill and also creates a vital pressure within the trunk.

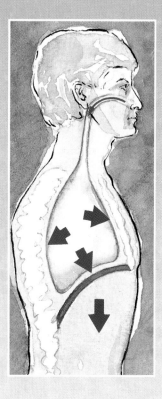

As you breathe out, the dome becomes more pronounced again and the pressure is released. This is the essential stimulus both for energy and the natural functioning of the whole of the trunk.

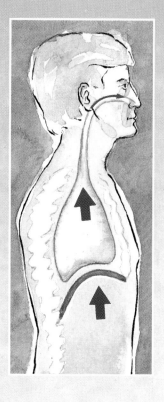

You can enhance this natural breathing process and benefit from it accordingly. Lying down is useful, because it makes the process easier, but the same action can be carried out sitting erect.

Place the heels of the hands to the sides of the rib-cage, against the bottom ribs. Concentrate on this area alone and, when you breathe in, let the ribs move out. As you begin to breathe out, firmly without jerking, press the ribs inwards. If they are stiff, be careful but persist steadily. Only if a rib has recently been cracked or damaged is there likely to be any problem. The flexibility of these ribs is an important element of our energy, mental and physical. Continue the squeeze-and-release process for up to five minutes and then take the hands away and relax for a minute or two before getting up.

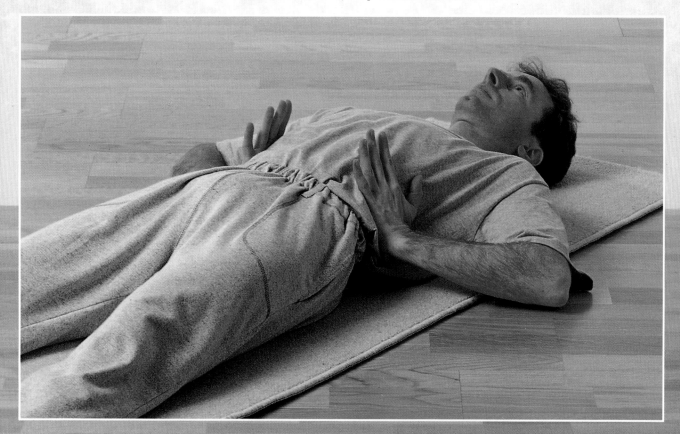

ABDOMINAL TONING

In addition to creating a strong, flexible spine, the abdominal muscles must be kept in good condition. Natural abdominal control is essential for effective breathing and it also keeps the glands and organs in good condition.

2

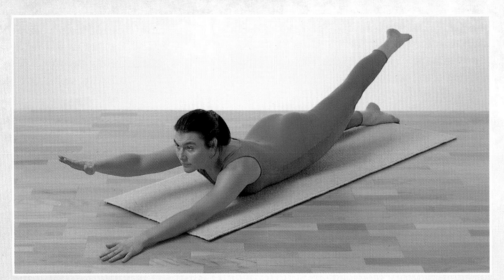

1 **The Canoe.** Lie on your front, chin against the floor, arms stretched in front, and with the feet close together.

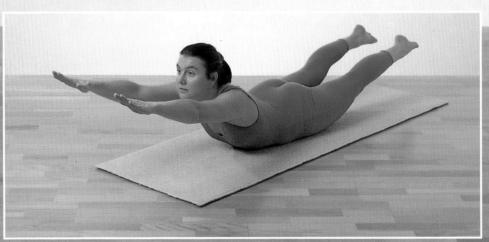

2 Having breathed out, stretch up the right arm and the left leg as you breathe in. Bring them down as you breathe out. Now repeat with the left arm and right leg. Perform each movement three times.

3 Finally, deepen the breathing a little and, as you breathe in, stretch up both arms and both legs, resting on the abdomen. Repeat this three times. Relax for a minute or two when you have finished.

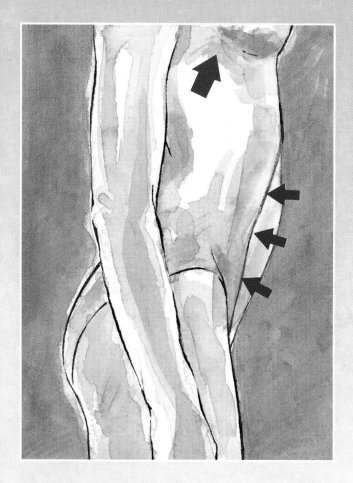

The abdominal muscles can be strengthened by breathing sharply out and, at the same time, pulling the muscles in. Relax them on the in-breath. This can be repeated a number of times. It will help as a preliminary for the Reverse Canoe posture.

UNDERSTANDING RHYTHM

Human life is a series of rhythms. When we are in good mental and physical health, these rhythms harmonize, like the different sections of a symphony orchestra. When they become discordant, when rhythm is lost, we suffer disease (literally, dis-ease), and when we are out of ease, mental and physical difficulties arise. Postures such as those on these pages should be seen from this point of view, not as mere exercises.

The Reverse Canoe.

Lying on your back, feet together, stretch the arms on the floor over your head, bringing the palms together. After breathing out, breathe in and raise the arms, head shoulders and legs. Do not bring the hands or feet more than about 40 cm (15 in) from the floor. This will maximize the tension on the abdominal muscles. Breathe out as you come down – slowly. Repeat three times, and then relax for a minute or two.

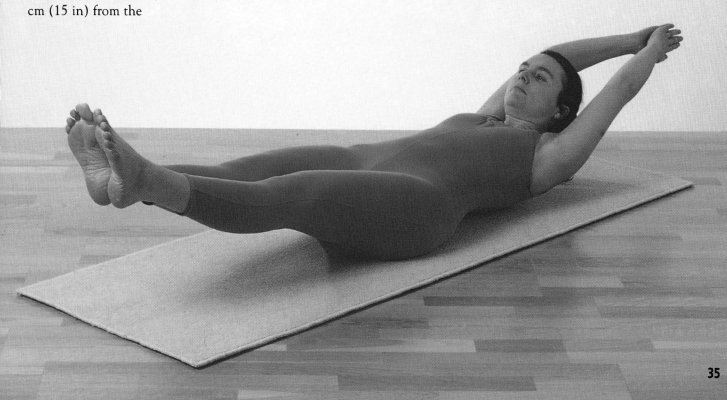

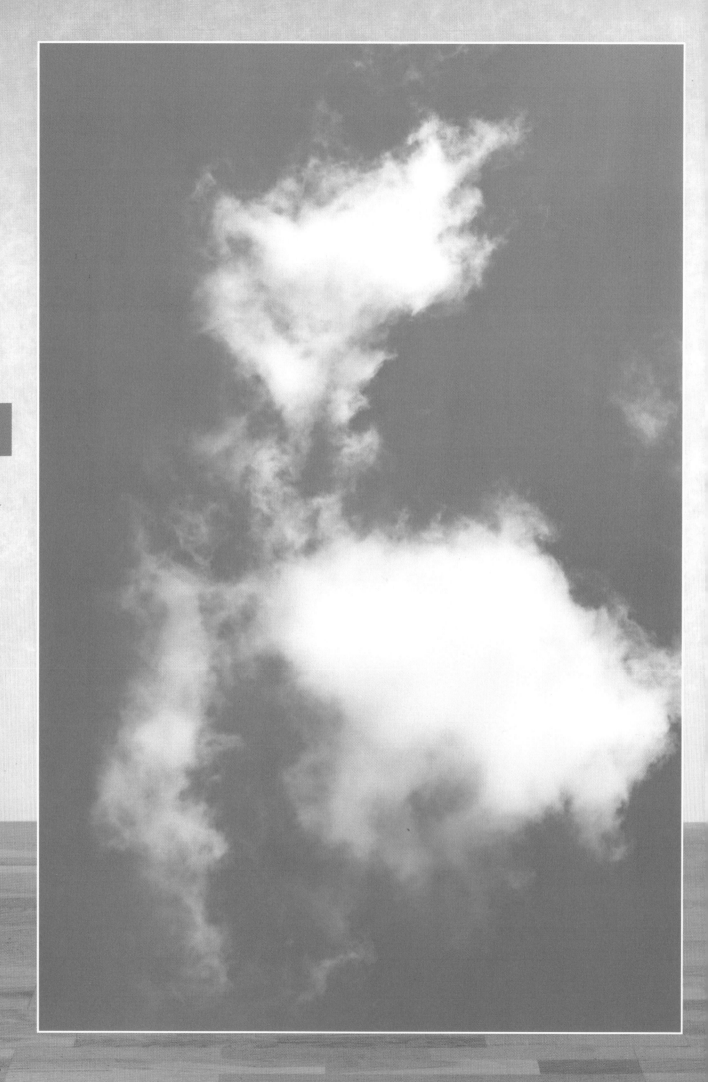

THE PROCESS OF VISUALIZATION

Visualization is a central aspect of human life; we conjure up pictures in our mind's eye all day long. Yoga trains us to take advantage of this natural phenomenon. If applied with concentration, the mind has amazing strength, but, if you simply play about with the idea, results will be only intermittent and unsatisfactory. The ability to retain a simple mental picture can be one of the most important achievements of life. A celebrated Indian yogi, Swami Rama, was involved in experiments at the Menninger Institute in America, where he showed he could control the beat of his heart by visualization.

CONTROLLING THOUGHT

A well-known swami once declared: "Human beings will do anything to help themselves – except to work for it." Once you realize that visualization is a natural, inbuilt process, you can determine to make it a part of your life. Of course, the brain will keep interposing irrelevant thoughts, but as you persist this will happen less and less. Once you have gained substantial mental control, your life will be enhanced tremendously.

2

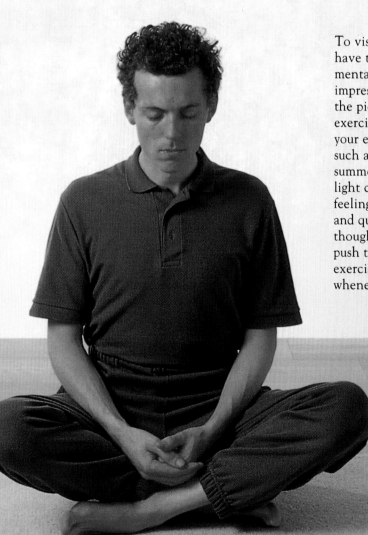

Swami Rama simply visualized a blue sky, with small, fluffy almost motionless clouds in it. Because his concentration was complete, the brain accepted this concept as reality and the whole body slowed down accordingly.

To visualize you do not have to create an actual mental picture, but an impression; the feeling of the picture. Simply as an exercise, sit erect, close your eyes and imagine such a sky: a beautiful summer's day, just a few light clouds and the feeling of peace, warmth and quiet. If other thoughts intrude, *gently* push them away. This exercise can be repeated whenever you feel like it.

THE RULES OF VISUALIZATION

To visualize effectively, remember that the human framework has developed very specifically. When sitting, we balance on the spine and the muscles need to be harmonized. The spine, too, is important for the working of the nervous system. It is not possible to visualize effectively if you slouch or if the trunk is distorted.

2

1 Unless you can already sit comfortably and correctly on the floor, use a chair. Do not rest against the chair-back unless it is upright. Close your eyes, and allow the head to balance comfortably on the shoulders. Wriggle the shoulders a little to ease any tension. Bring the hands together on the lap. Listen to the gentle sound of your breath: feel the cool touch of air on your nostrils as you breathe in and the warm flow of air as you breathe out. Feel the sense of relaxation as you breathe out.

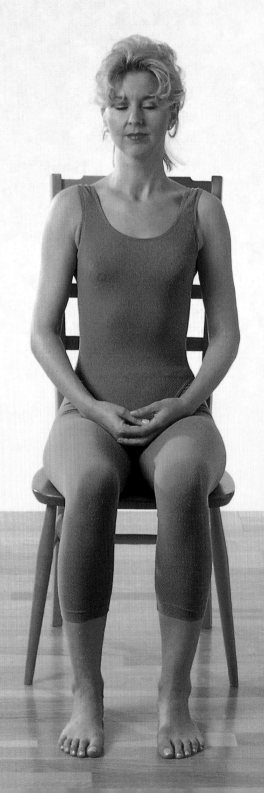

2 Time is now irrelevant. The slow rhythm of your breath is like the comforting tick of a grandfather clock – it enhances the stillness, rather than detracts from it. As you breathe out, repeat to yourself, "I am at peace". When you are truly at ease, gently begin to bring in the visualization you have decided upon. Establish the feeling of it; let it flow all around you. This is to become your reality: you have gone into your own world and are now living fully in it.

A SIMPLE VISUALIZATION

Each breath we take is an intake of energy –
not just from the flow of oxygen through the
lungs, but by the stimulation of the body's
electro-magnetic force. In yoga, this is known
as prana. It flows through the nervous
system, stimulates the constant reinforcement
of bone tissue, controls the heartbeat and
passes messages through the brain. Every cell
in the body has its own electrical field, while
the diaphragm acts as the pump of the
whole system.

Sitting quietly, having checked your posture,
concentrate on your breathing, making it
slow, rhythmical and peaceful. Visualize your
breath as you draw it in through your nostrils
as a warm, soothing mist spreading as a
warming flow up to the top of the head.
Breathing slowly out, feel the breath flow
through every part of your body, down to the
tips of the toes. If any other thought intrudes,
quietly push it away and let this picture
become totally real to you.

Continue for a minimum of five minutes
(in due course, anything up to 20 minutes).
As you finish, let the visualization fade away,
retaining the feeling of warming energy.
Open your eyes and stretch.

In the early stages of
visualization you can get
into the right mood by
recalling a time when
everything felt good.
A holiday, perhaps,
where the sense of peace
and the warmth of the
sun united to make you
feel totally in harmony.
Such recollections can
help you create your
own images.

2

DEVISING A PROGRAMME

It is important to integrate the various facets of yoga practice into the daily routine of life. Some people say, "I can't afford the time". The reply is: "You can't afford not to".

A major benefit of yoga discipline is that it makes you feel good. That feeling helps the body in all its activities and also makes the mind clearer and more incisive. Half-an-hour spent giving yourself to these practices will save at least a full hour of muddle and stressed activities.

The need for regular practice is not confined to the postures. Helping breathing, calming the mind, promoting peace and health, all have a central role to play.

There is much to be said for setting aside a specific time each day for practice, but if this is not possible, then at least try to fit the activities into any time that is available, provided that you allow at least 1½ hours to digest a small snack or two hours for a meal before you begin. This applies to the breathing and mental practices as well as the postures. Allowing digestion to proceed unhampered is important.

POSTURES
Stretching and relaxing forms an important preliminary to practising postures. Stretching should always be counter-balanced by the relaxed swing. Neck and shoulder exercises should be performed in every session.

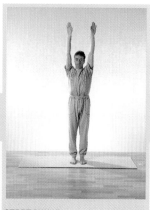

STRETCHING   Page 22

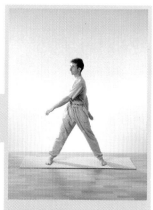

STRETCHING   Page 22

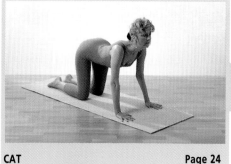

CAT   Page 24

The Cat and the simple Spinal Twist provide important toning and enhance flexibility of the spine. Especially in the early stages, these should be the first spinal movements undertaken.

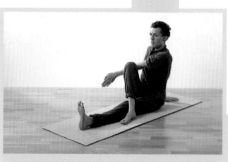

SPINAL TWIST   Page 25

The Back Body Stretch lifts the trunk to elongate the spine. Avoid a humpy bend as you stretch forward, but equally ease the back into stretching. Then, with the Cobra, ensure you balance the arms and trunk, so the back can relax without any sense of strain.

2

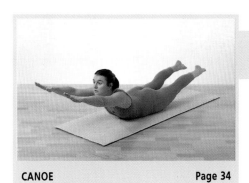

CANOE Page 34

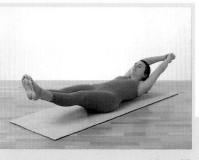

REVERSE CANOE Page 35

RELAXATION
Relax for at least a minute between all postures which demand the holding of muscle tension. At the end of a posture session, relax for at least five minutes. Most yoga sessions conclude with a relaxation of around 15 minutes.

2

The Canoe and the Reverse Canoe will tone the abdominal muscles. In the Canoe, legs and arms stretch upwards (as shown); in the Reverse Canoe the limits indicated should be followed. In the early stages, watch yourself in a mirror, until you know you are doing it correctly.

BREATHING
Both during a posture session and during the day, pay attention to harmonizing the breath. Ease the rib cage into flexibility, enjoy seeing that your breathing is rhythmical. Be aware of the whole process of energization.

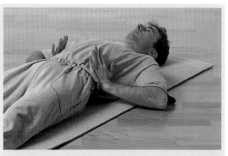

RELAXATION Page 31

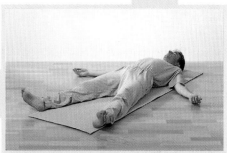

Page 33

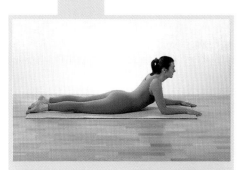

COBRA Page 29

VISUALIZATION
As with breathing, visualization should play a role throughout the day. Do not dwell on the stressful aspects of life – although this does not mean ignoring them altogether – instead promote thoughts of harmony, peace and beauty. Mind and body will respond.

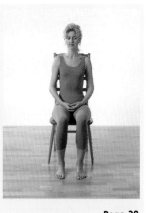

Page 38

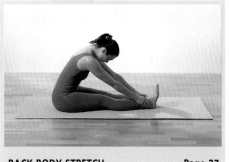

BACK BODY STRETCH Page 27

MINUTE·BY·MINUTE
YOGA

AIMS FOR THE MONTH

The practice of yoga is not merely setting time aside regularly for exercising or relaxation. It is a total approach to living. There is little value in setting brief periods aside for beneficial activities if you slip back into old bad habits the rest of the time. In months 1 and 2, the total interconnection between mind and body has been emphasized. Now that you have practised some basic movements and glimpsed the exciting mental potential, you can take this integration further.

RELAXING AT HOME

The word "relax" is often used in two different senses. The yoga sense is letting-go by correct use of mind and body; the everyday sense is to flop out. We may not say, "Let's slouch in front of the television", but that is what we do. At meals, also, we all too often hunch our shoulders and crush our digestive system.

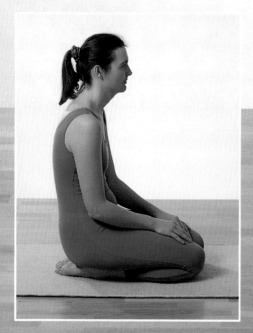

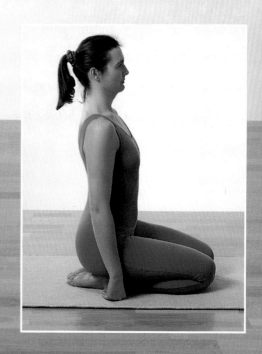

1 Slouching is depleting: back muscles are affected, breathing impaired and the functioning of digestion and the abdominal organs impeded.

2 Sitting with a thrust-out chest also affects back muscles, can all too easily impede the nervous system, and results in shallow and ineffectual breathing.

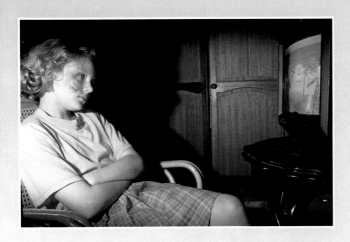

Naturally, no one needs to sit correctly *all* the time, but to be effectively active or pleasantly relaxed correct posture is important. The art of sitting correctly has been a central point of yoga for thousands of years, not just as a discipline, but to allow us make the most of both body and mind. Many problems can stem – or develop – from "flopped out" evenings.

3

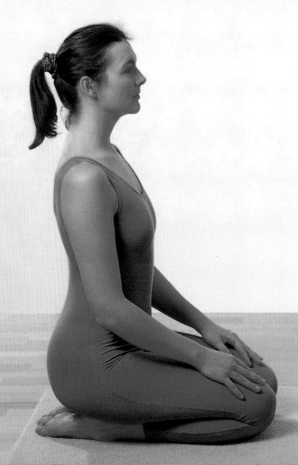

3 The need for an upright, but not rigid, posture cannot be over-emphasized. These pictures are posed in a simple sitting position, but chairs, sensibly used, are just as effective. Sitting well, you are both more mentally alert and are using the body healthily.

MOVING UPSIDE-DOWN

*T*he one thing that most people know about
yoga is that practitioners often stand on their
heads! The Head Stand is not included in this
programme because it needs careful teaching
and, if self-taught, can be harmful. Other
inverted positions are easier to learn, and do
provide real benefits. The Half-shoulder
Stand, for example, improves circulation and
blood flow, stimulates the thyroid gland and –
when performed in a relaxed manner – takes
pressure off the heart.

3

**1 The Half-shoulder
Stand.** Lie on your
back, legs together and
hands by the sides, palms
down. Remember the
shoulders will take much
of the weight, so make
sure they are not tense –
wriggle them firmly
before beginning. Be
aware, too, that you will
achieve the position
with a comfortable swing
from a relaxed body.

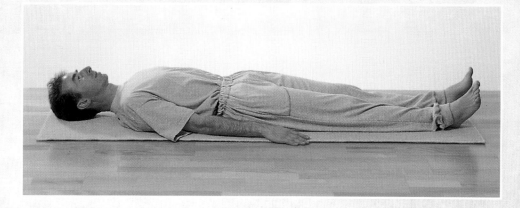

2 Having breathed out,
breathe in, swinging
the legs *and trunk* into
the air (legs either bent
or straight) as though
you were going to roll
over on your back.

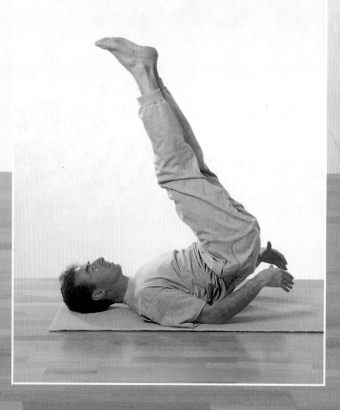

4 Coming down, use an out-breath, bring the arms, palms down, on the floor behind you to take the weight and *slowly* lower the legs, again, either bent or straight. As the body becomes balanced in each aspect of the *asana*, the whole position becomes both stimulating and peaceful. When you have completed the posture, relax totally for a minute or two.

IMPROVING BODY AWARENESS

The Half- and Full-shoulder Stands are excellent postures for improving awareness of the body. As youngsters we loved to roll on our backs, and we need to recapture this exuberance. A major reason why children have such energy is that they let it flow freely. Adults tend to block or deplete it. The Shoulder Stand, properly performed, is a great energizer.

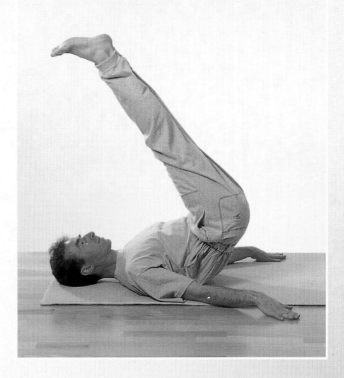

3 As the legs reach a vertical position, let the hands lightly hold the small of the back. Feel the shoulders rather than the back of the neck taking the pressure. Stretch the toes into the air and then relax the feet. Breathe slowly and rhythmically. Initially, hold for, say, 30 seconds. You will be able to increase this time substantially with practice.

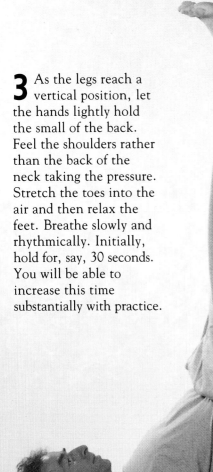

THE FISH

This is the counter-pose to the Half-shoulder Stand, since it compresses the cervical vertibrae after they have been extended. It also opens the chest fully.

1 Lying on the floor with the feet together, raise the trunk on the elbows, arching the back and letting the head drop back.

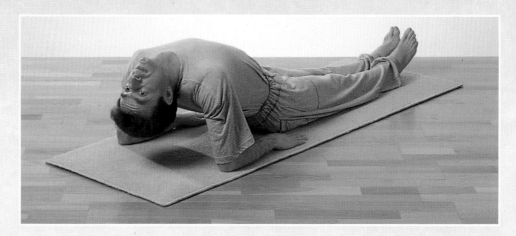

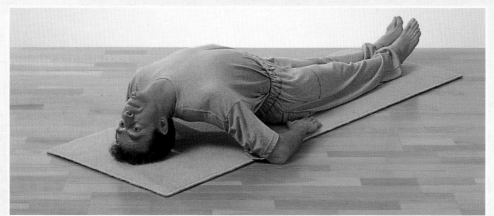

2 Move the elbows so that the crown of the head rests on the floor and the chest is expanded.

3 Bring the palms of the hands together on the chest in the prayer *(namaste)* position. Breathe slowly and deeply. Hold for about 30 seconds.

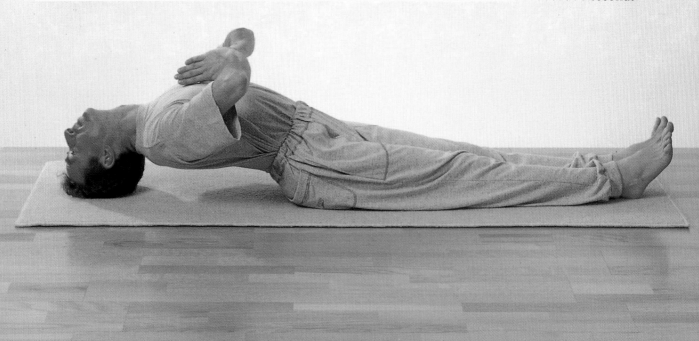

VISUALIZATION IN THE POSTURES

The asanas *largely developed from meditative practices. If you hold or use the body in a balanced position and then let your mind dwell on some beneficial concept, the body will naturally adapt itself, becoming more free and supple. This is not easy to achieve, but it brings great benefits. It is one of the unique aspects of yoga, setting it apart from other approaches.*

Regular practice of the postures will ensure *that they are performed with the minimum tension and with no waste of energy. As this happens, the visualization aspect can be introduced. Some of the postures you have been practising should now be coming along well. When you are holding those that feel comfortable and balanced, let your mind dwell on a beautiful sunrise and experience that wonderful sensation of well-being it evokes. You will find that you can hold the posture better and it will be comfortable for longer.*

Always work with ideas that you find comfortable. For most people a beautiful dawn is inspiring, but a few may have had an unhappy experience that it could awaken. If so, choose another image. Remember, making progress in yoga is a two-way process. Absorb what you are taught, but never forget that you have your own role to play.

3

TAKING STOCK

It is now time to pause and reflect on the progress to date, as well as considering the next steps. Each month has contained some new asanas, but you may well wish that more had been included. The classical language that the sages of yoga used was Sanscrit.
It contains a beautiful word: santosha.
This means being content with where you are and building on that contentment.
It does not mean "putting up with" but rather "working from".

Most people embark upon the path of yoga because they want to enhance their life. Everyone needs thoughts to inspire them. For many centuries the sages of yoga have likened human life to the growth of the Lotus flower or Water Lily. The flower is one of the most perfect there is: a circle of beautiful petals glowing on the top of the water of the lake. The Buddhists have a beautiful saying: *"Om mane padme hum"* – "Behold the jewel in the flower of the Lotus". The root of the Lotus, however, is deep in slimey mud at the bottom of the lake. The Lotus root uses these murky ingredients as its nutrients and sends out shoots, which rise in the water until they breast the surface. There – and only there – the bud forms and the perfect flower emerges.

Our lives and the Lotus
Especially in these days of turmoil, our own lives, like the Lotus roots, seem to be submerged and it is easy for us to think that we cannot rise above the problems which surround us. The difficulties and problems that weigh us down are challenges to be faced and overcome, like the Lotus, we can send up shoots that will eventually bloom in the sunshine.

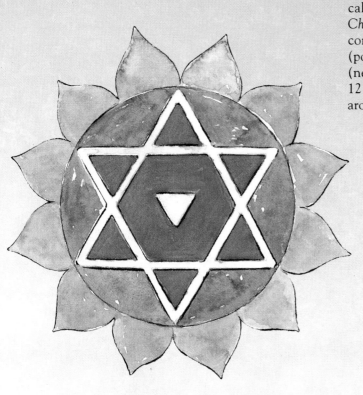

The Heart Centre is called the *Anahata Chakra* in Sanskrit. It combines the sun (positive) and the moon (negative) symbols, with 12 Lotus Flower petals around it.

CONCENTRATION

These days we are all too often told we can master important things with very little effort. This is just not true. We can ease the learning process a little but we need *santosha*, and this depends upon developing the power of concentration. Concentration is often talked about and advocated, but few people have the slightest idea of how to achieve it. The specific suggestions offered will help but "If at first we don't succeed..."

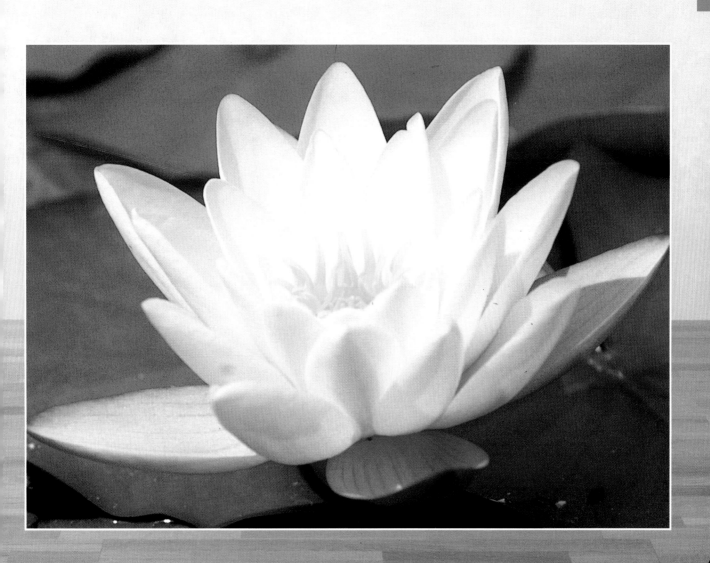

CONTINUING THE PROGRAMME

As you get used to practising the yoga postures, see that your understanding of them deepens. It is all too easy to slip into a routine of doing them automatically and thoughtlessly, whereas the exact opposite is essential. Progress comes from "going with" the posture, not from creating the wrong tensions, whether mental or physical. The often-made statement that yoga is not competitive does not infer that your attitude to its performance is unconsidered; in other words, creating harmony of mind, body and energy produces the finest results.

3

POSTURES
By now you will notice that even simple movements, like these stretches, produce deeper results. As a dog's body expresses happiness when it is taken for a walk, so the body shows its joy at being effectively stretched.

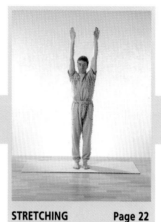

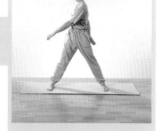

STRETCHING   Page 22

STRETCHING   Page 22

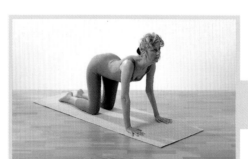

CAT   Page 24

You also become increasingly aware of the benefit of counter-balancing postures. A stretch forwards is always matched with a stretch backwards and so on, as shown here.

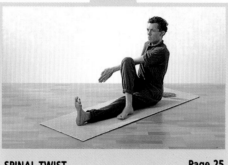

SPINAL TWIST   Page 25

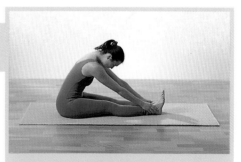

BACK BODY STRETCH   Page 27

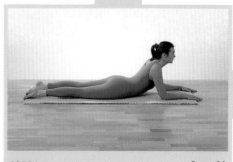

COBRA   Page 29

RELAXATION
Remember to follow a session of postures with a minimum of five minutes relaxation.

BREATHING AND VISUALIZATION
Separate breathing activity is important, but visualization interlocks mind and breath.

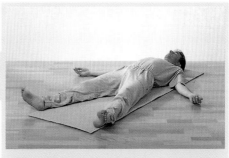

RELAXATION   **Page 31**

Correct posture (as shown here) brings many benefits, headed by the balancing of the nervous system, which plays such an important role in life.

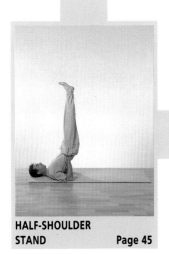

HALF-SHOULDER STAND   **Page 45**

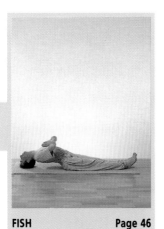

FISH   **Page 46**

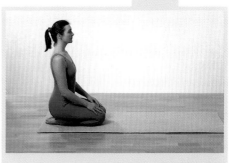

Page 43

You see this counter-balance when you begin to feel the benefits of inversion. The contrasted

activities of neck and shoulders in the following two postures provide an excellent case in point.

Harmonious and rhythmical breathing leads you towards harmonious and rhythmical thoughts – the core of visualization.

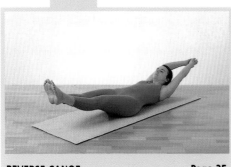

REVERSE CANOE   **Page 35**

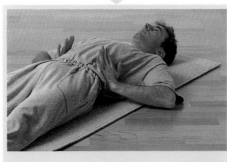

Page 33

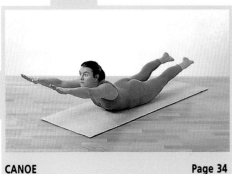

CANOE   **Page 34**

In addition to the practice of enhancing the breath while lying on your back, practice in a sitting position can be introduced at almost any time of the day, with good results.

MEDITATION

AIMS FOR THE MONTH

The four complementary aspects of human life are activation, relaxation, visualization and meditation. All are essential to a truly fulfilled existence; all are the basic weapons of health and happiness. You are now using your body in association with the mind and the energy through the breath. You are stimulating your life through relaxation and visualization. Incorporating the peace of meditation is the next major step. In this month you practise more asanas, but, even more importantly, deepen the way in which you use your body, not only when practising yoga, but also in all aspects of life.

. . . .

FIRST STEPS

What are the differences between relaxation, visualization and meditation? In relaxation you allow the body to tick over, like an idling engine, while you observe but do not interfere. In visualization, you use imagery to stimulate the functioning of the body. In meditation you withdraw the mind from the body (without losing awareness of its presence) and dwell on a single, non-physical concept. This takes you beyond the normal limitations of living, to achieve a much greater sense of control.

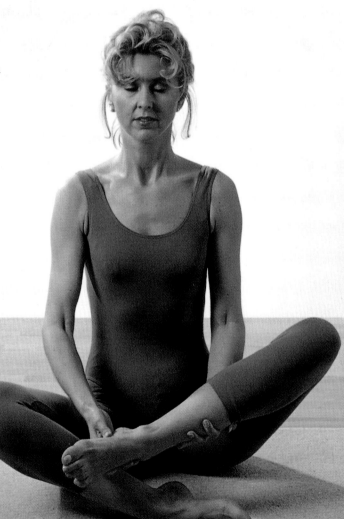

You can meditate sitting either in a chair or on the floor. It is not practical to meditate lying down. The conditions already explained (see pages 28–29) apply here: the trunk must be comfortably upright, the hands together (or in a more classical position, in which thumb and forefinger of each hand are touching) and the eyes closed. Some schools advocate meditation with the eyes half-open, but most people find this extremely difficult. It is essential that the body should be comfortable, otherwise messages of distress are signalled to the brain and the calm mental basis is impossible.

There are countless ways of meditating and it is sensible to try several to find one that really suits you, but do not flutter about like a butterfly; that will not be helpful.

Hamsa meditation

An image that has been used for centuries in Indian meditation is that of the wild goose or swan. These creatures are equally at home on land, water or in the air. As such, they have come to symbolize the free spirit. An effective way to begin meditating is to sit correctly in a room where you will not be disturbed. Close your eyes and bring your mind to the flow and sound of your breath. After a minute or two visualize a goose or swan flying through the air. The Sanscrit word for the bird is *Hamsa*. Keep the visualization for a few minutes and then, as you breathe in, repeat to yourself, "Ham", as you breathe out, repeat "sa". "Ham . . . sa".

Now let the vision of the bird fade, but continue to repeat "Ham . . . sa" together with the in- and out-breath. Any stray thoughts which intrude should be gently pushed away and the chanting resumed. Initially, around ten minutes is long enough. Gradually you can extend this and, before long, between 20 and 30 minutes will become ideal.

As you get more used to the practice, you will not only find that your mind is both peaceful and alert, but your body will also feel lithe and supple, for the physical benefits of meditation are considerable.

4

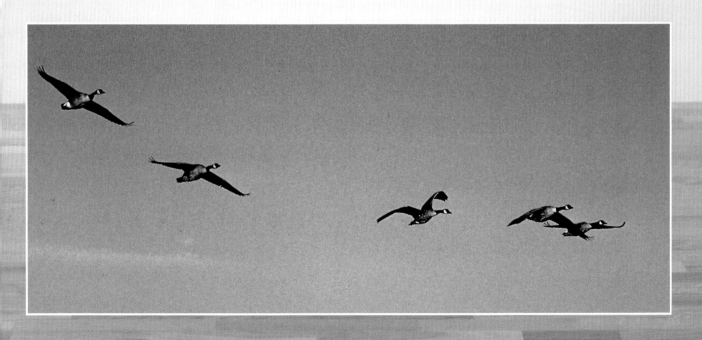

THE MOUNTAIN BREATH

Initially, we have concentrated on enhancing the natural process of breathing, because all too often the pressures and style of daily living have damaged the way we breathe. Now you can practise a few techniques that will benefit both body and breath, and stimulate the flow of energy. The first of these, the Mountain Breath, reminds us that the atmosphere in mountainous regions and areas with rushing streams is more highly charged with negative ions, that have been found to be beneficial both mentally and physically.

1 Stand, or sit, comfortably erect, with the arms by the sides. Be aware you are standing tall. Breathe out slowly.

2 As you breathe in, stretch the arms, raising them to the sides, a little behind the line of the shoulders, so that, as they come up, the muscles of the trunk are stretched and lifted.

3 When you have stretched up fully, link the thumbs and hold the air in the lungs. After some seconds, begin to breathe out, bringing the arms down, maintaining the stretch. Repeat the exercise at least five times.

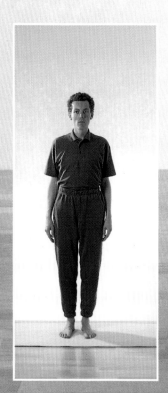

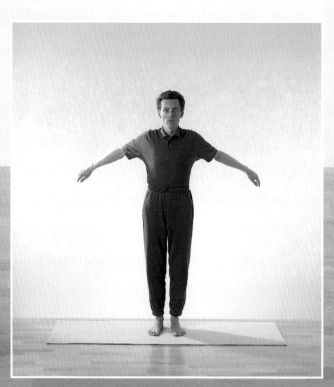

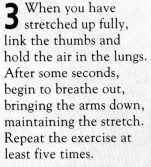

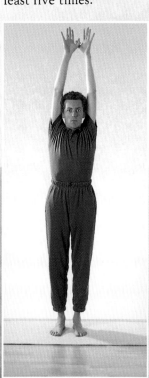

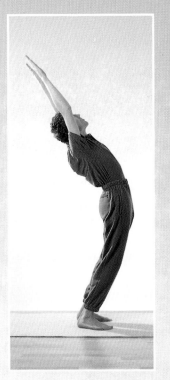

1 Cleansing Breath.
In these sedentary times, people's breathing is often shallow, and stale air collects in the bottom of the lungs. Offset this by standing erect, feet a little apart, then swing the arms up, bending back a little, mouth closed.

2 Now swing right forward, breathing out through the mouth with a strong "Ha" sound. The head should be loose and the arms dangling. Pull in the abdominal muscles to get more air out of the lungs. Repeat three times.

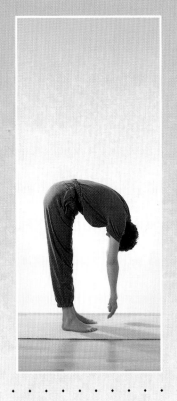

EXPERIENCING PRANA

It is all too easy to underestimate the importance of the breath. Literally it *is* life and should be revered as such. When concentrating on the breath – whether to enhance it naturally or by means of specific exercises – the mind should wonder at this Life Force, called in yoga *prana*.

LUNG CLEARING BREATH

LUNG CLEARING BREATH

Pollution, smoking and shallow breathing all tend to clog the passages of the lungs, as X-ray pictures show. This exercise squeezes the full lungs to help dislodge mucus and blockages. Anyone with severe chest problems or emphysema should consult their physician before practising it.

1 Standing as for the Mountain, breathe in, stretching out the arms, bend the elbows and place the fingers on the tops of the shoulder.

2 Retaining the breath, and keeping the fingers on the shoulders bring the elbows to the front.

3 Drop the head and bend forward from the waist, squeezing the chest, still with the breath retained. Hold for several seconds. Then come up breathing out and reverse the initial movement. Repeat three times.

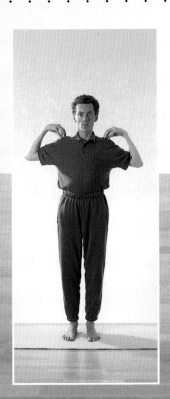

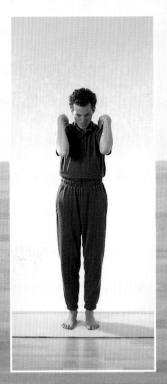

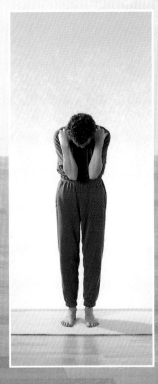

UPSIDE-DOWN AGAIN

Is it natural to up-end ourselves? You have
only to look at children playing to get the
answer – they love cartwheels, handstands
and rolling over and over. Keeping the body
active and even turning it upside-down is a
naturally inherited instinct. The inverted
positions of yoga rationalize this instinct, to
our mental and physical benefit. The Pose of
Tranquility is a topsy-turvy posture that is
physically stimulating and mentally calming.
While yoga asanas are performed with
control, the swing and sense of balance we all
had as uninhibited children are essential to
effective performance.

1 Pose of Tranquility.
Lie on the floor, feet
together, arms by the
sides, palms down.
Breathe quite deeply
and, on an in-breath,
swing the legs into the
air, using arms and
hands to provide both
pressure and balance.

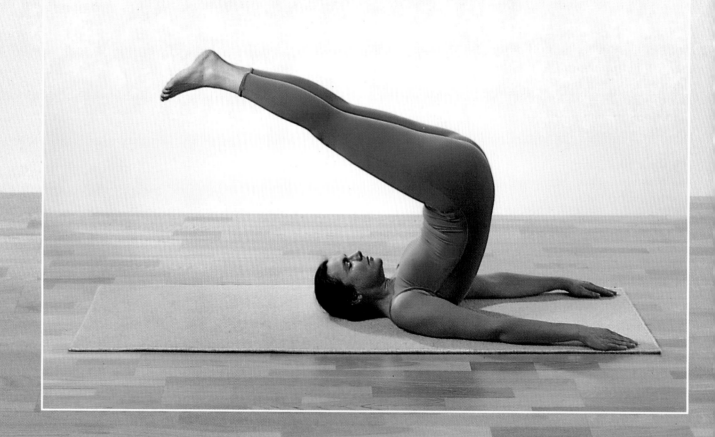

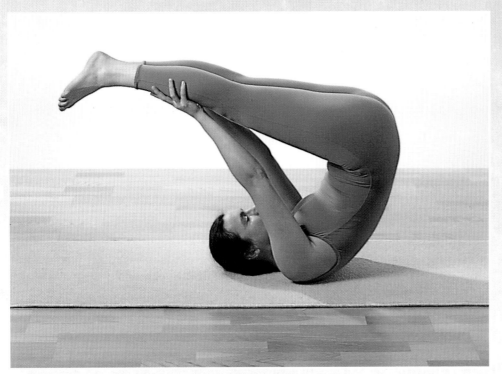

REGAINING CHILDISH ZEST

Getting back childish zest is an important aspect of adult practice: you need to combine that instinct with thoughtfulness. While the slow, controlled performance is central to yoga, you can often make progress by first of all coming back to the roll-about aspect of childhood and, from this, impose the greater control learned as an adult.

2 When you feel balanced on the shoulders, bring up the arms and hold ankles or shins. The arms are straight, not bent at the elbows. Retain the position, preferably with the eyes closed, breathing gently. Gradually develop a floating feeling. Hold it for as long as is comfortable. Bring the arms back to the floor first to control the slow lowering of the legs.

3 The Plough. From the Pose of Tranquility, you can move into The Plough (so-called because the body resembles a horse-drawn plough). Remove the hands from the legs, lowering the legs until the toes touch the floor. Maintain balance by letting the fingers lightly support the back. As with the Pose of Tranquility, when coming down, bring the arms to the floor first and use them to control the slow movement of the legs. Relax for a minute or two.

4

CONTROLLING OUR RESPONSES

Life is a series of challenges and how people meet these will over the years play a major role in their outlook and health. It has been shown that happy events can challenge people as much as unhappy ones; all are aspects of that much-used word, stress. No one can avoid stressful events, but it is possible to control reactions to them. Classically, yoga texts urge that both happy and unhappy events be treated with dispassion. Few will achieve this, but it is not difficult to bring about beneficial modifications.

1 Bad news affects breathing, which in turn seizes up the muscles of the trunk. The flow of energy to the brain, too, is impaired, making clear thinking difficult. If something bad happens, sit quietly, place the hands on the chest, deliberately slow your breathing and be aware of your control both of breathing in and breathing out. In a minute or two you will feel the pressure ease.

2 Even good news can upset your equilibrium. To accept good news calmly and effectively, bring the hands, palms downwards at chest level and feel you are pushing down the gasping sensation which arises. Let the hands rise a little as you breathe in and descend slowly on the out breath. Again, ensure that the breath is slowed.

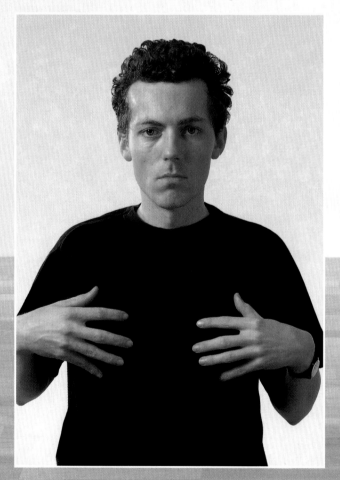

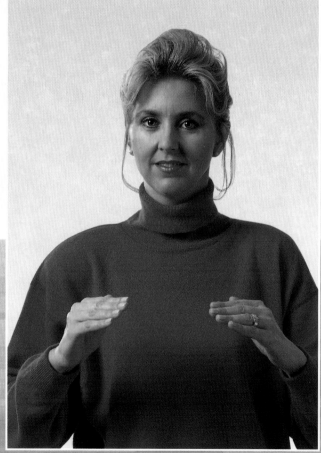

CHANGING

Reactions to life events become firm reflexes and are hard to change. But change *is* possible and where these reactions are damaging – which is all too often the case – it is important to work to bring it about. For example, the rushing person, always looking at his or her watch and dashing from one thing to the next, can be helped by simply sticking a little coloured circle on the watch-face. Every time the watch is looked at there is a reminder of the need to slow down.

3 If something causes worry, you tend to feel that your head is spinning and that you can't quite grasp what is going on. As with all these emotions, conscious slowing and quieting of the breath is essential and, in this case, placing the fingertips gently on the forehead helps to reduce the mental turmoil.

4 Irritating or annoying news can, if not checked, lead to harmful reactions. Bringing the hands on to the chest in the prayer position (*namaste*) has a calming effect, just by its body language. Encourage the breathing to slow and the annoyance will abate.

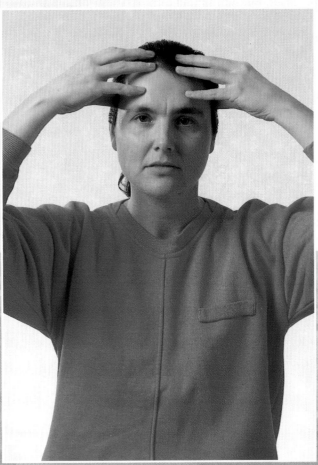

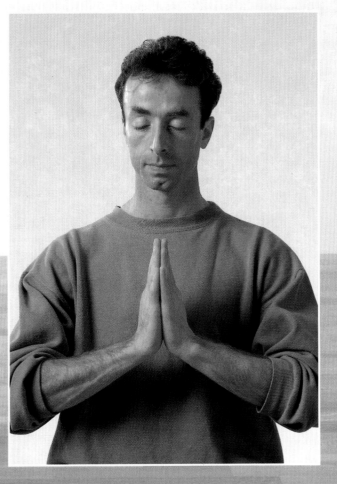

59

CONTINUING THE PROGRAMME

A scientific law, which is also at the heart of yoga thinking, runs as follows: nothing is created, nothing is destroyed, everything is in the process of changing. Any yoga programme, too, needs to develop, mature and change. The emphasis this month moves specifically to the breath. It by no means ignores the postures, but it explores the remarkable enhancement to life that effective control of respiration can bring.

While visualization now plays an important daily role in life, you can begin to explore the wonders of meditation. "Wonders" is, indeed, the word, for meditation can lift you to hitherto undreamed of realms – providing you take it slowly, do not expect miracles, and allow it to develop at its own pace.

BREATHING
However well you advance in yoga, there will always be a place for controlling the breath with the use of the hands.

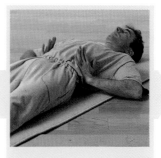

Page 33

The Mountain Posture combines strong use of the body with valuable development of breathing and this can be linked with the "Ha" breath.

Keeping the lungs clear is of value to everyone, not just those afflicted by chest complaints.

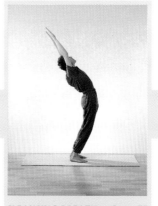

CLEANSING BREATH   Page 55

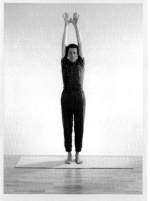

MOUNTAIN BREATH   Page 54

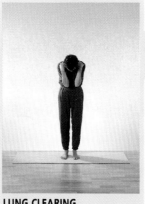

LUNG CLEARING BREATH   Page 55

Using these guidelines, you should now be able to devise a breathing sequence of, say, ten minutes, which will help you in every way.

POSTURES
Practising a sequence of balanced postures, such as that shown here, will make body, energy and mind respond. Such a session, even if it is no more than 15 or 20 minutes will leave you glowing.

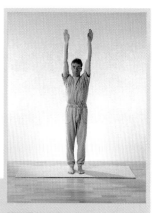

STRETCHING   Page 22

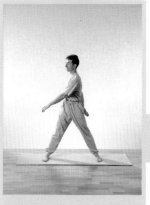

STRETCHING   Page 22

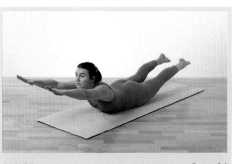

CANOE   **Page 34**

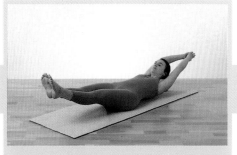

REVERSE CANOE   **Page 35**

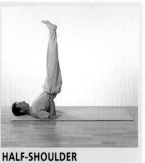

HALF-SHOULDER STAND   **Page 45**

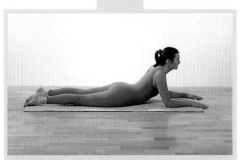

COBRA   **Page 29**

In some ways the Plough is the most demanding pose so far. Its successful performance comes not from striving but from allowing it to happen.

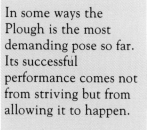

FISH   **Page 46**

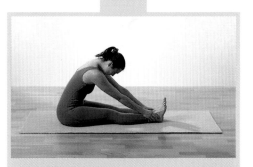

BACK BODY STRETCH   **Page 27**

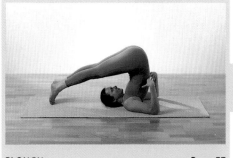

PLOUGH   **Page 57**

RELAXATION
The final relaxation is becoming more and more important as your physical *asanas* become more demanding.

4

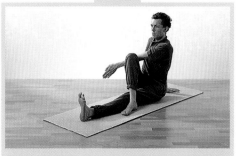

SPINAL TWIST   **Page 25**

MEDITATION
Many people are scared of meditation, yet it is a totally natural process. Neither snatch at it nor be afraid of it.

Initially, just feel the joy of letting both body and brain calm down and function quietly.

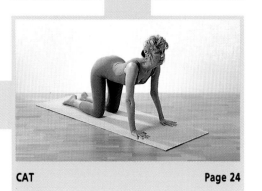

CAT   **Page 24**

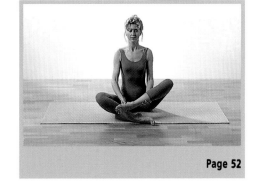

Page 52

5

BODY AND MIND

AIMS FOR THE MONTH

People taking up yoga start with a variety of different physical conditions. However, the majority begin with stiffness and some ideas of major limitations. One thing is clear: the body responds to intelligent use. This month you can work a little more deeply towards psychophysical balance. The way you enter into the performance of the asanas will play a major role in determining how well you succeed. It is a good idea to visualize trees and bushes responding to the wind. The graceful movement of the branches suggests a willingness to go with the force.

THE BRIDGE

All postures based on spinal activity also benefit most other parts of the body. Rhythmical massaging of the abdominal organs, for instance, can arise from a combination of movement and breath. Such massage will play a major role in maintaining good health. Meanwhile, spinal flexibility can make a remarkable difference in freeing your body from potential damage.

1 Lie on your back, the arms by the side, palms down, and draw the heels into the buttocks. Breathe out.

2 As you breathe in, raise the back, buttocks and thighs and bring the hands into the small of the back, palms open, with the elbows helping to support you. Retain the breath and come back slowly on the out-breath when ready.

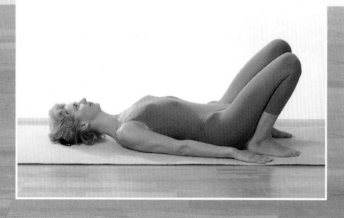

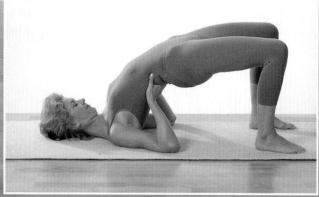

PROGRESS IN THE PLOUGH

Many yoga postures have variations, which provide a further benefit, but their performance is optional. This variation on the Plough position has the unfortunate name of the Choking Pose, but do not let that put you off. There is no need to choke and the development is beneficial!

• • • • • • • • • • • • • • • •

The Choking Pose

1 Move into the Plough as previously shown and hold the position for a minute or two breathing quietly. Do not be in any rush.

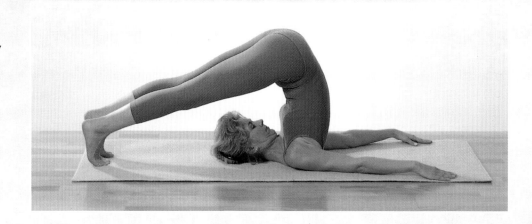

2 Then on an out-breath, bend the knees and bring them on to the floor by the shoulders. Bring the arms around and clasp the hands over the back of the knees by the crown of the head.

Again, hold the position calmly with a gentle breath. Come back into the normal Plough position when you feel ready and, finally, return to the floor slowly on a controlled out-breath. Relax.

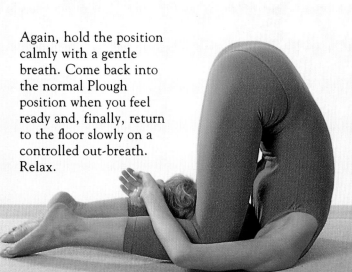

5

SIDEWAYS BEND

1 Stand, legs apart, palms against thighs.

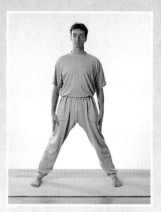

The four basic movements of the spine are forwards, backwards, sideways and twisting. The sideways movement is important, not only for the spine itself but also alternately to open up and compress each side of the chest and abdomen. At the same time, the mind, dwelling on reaching out to the right and then to the left, will be calmly focused, helping to improve physical and mental health.

2 As you breathe in, slowly stretch the right arm up, turning the palm inwards, until the arm is touching the ear.

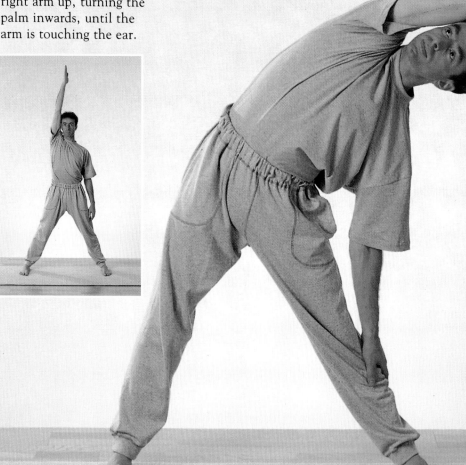

3 With the breath retained, stretch the arm up as high as it can go, lifting the shoulder. Breathing out, slowly bend to the left, arm still stretched, until the arm is parallel with the floor. Keep the shoulders parallel with the hips. Hold the position for at least 30 seconds, then reverse the movements and perform the posture with the left arm.

5

SPINAL TWIST (LEGS BENT)

Having performed the Spinal Twist with the leg stretched (see page 25), you can move on to a development in which both legs are bent. Each version of the posture has its own value.

Once you have assured yourself that you have got the physical details of postures right, performance depends almost entirely on your state of mind. Do not fuss about the body but dwell on simple, peaceful conceptions. Make sure these are still, or almost so; do not let your thoughts jump about.

1 From a sitting position on the floor, bend the right leg into the groin and bring the left leg over the right knee. The left palm is placed on the floor in line with the centre of the back but a few inches from it. Do not lean on the arm.

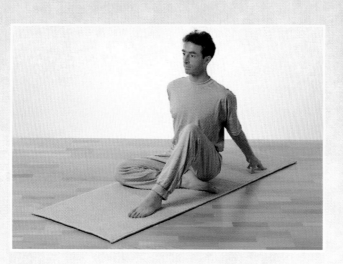

2 The right elbow comes across the bent left knee, cuddling it into the chest.

3 Breathe in. Then, as you breathe out, firmly twist the shoulders to the left. Keep balanced on each cheek of the bottom. Close your eyes and feel you are looking round at a beautiful, still scene. Hold for some two minutes, come slowly back to the original position and repeat on the other side.

5

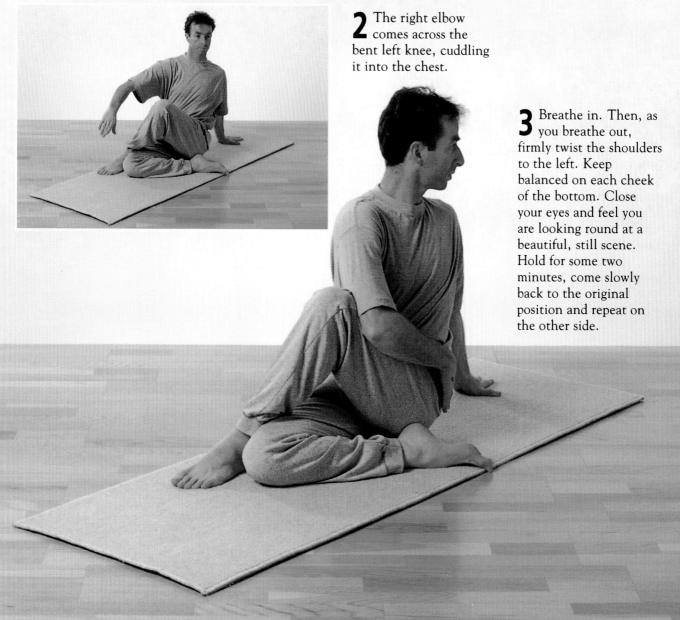

65

SPINAL PROGRESS

It is all too easy to continue to perform a posture regularly without making any mental or physical progress. Careful, slow progress is important. This is especially true of asanas, which are freeing parts of the body that all too easily seize up, especially the spine, the muscles of the trunk and the hamstrings.

Back Body Stretch.
Allowing the lower back to become rigid is all too common and leads to much suffering. Do not forget to lift the back as you come forward, but aim to maintain the stretch without maintaining a sense of tension. Above all, do not be concerned about time. If the mind is quiet and the breathing calm and controlled, the muscles and joints will adjust themselves.

5

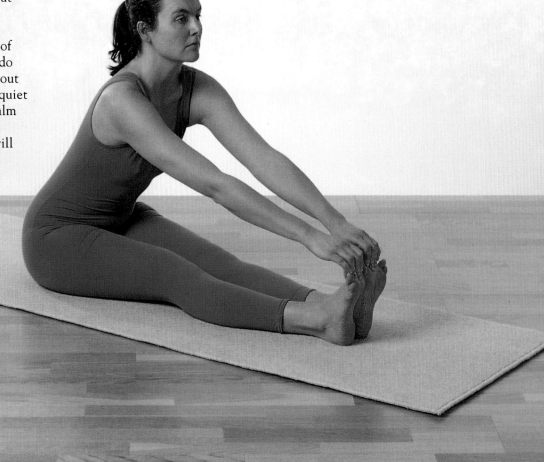

Here we take another look at the Back Body Stretch and the Cobra. If, with the Stretch, you have so far managed to hold the ankle or calf, now is the time to aim at reaching the toes. With the Cobra, the straight arms should move in closer, so the spine achieves a deeper curve. In each case, the progress is achieved by allowing it to happen, rather than by grim determination. To succeed, concentrate more completely and ensure that all external considerations are being eliminated.

· · · · · · · · · · · · · · · · ·

SPINAL PROGRESS

5

The Cobra. With the arms held straight (not bent at the elbows) the arms and trunk are balanced, so there is no undue pressure and the position can be held comfortably. Make quite sure the hips are on the floor, not coming up into the air. The compression in the lower back counters the stretch of the previous posture and strengthens the whole area.

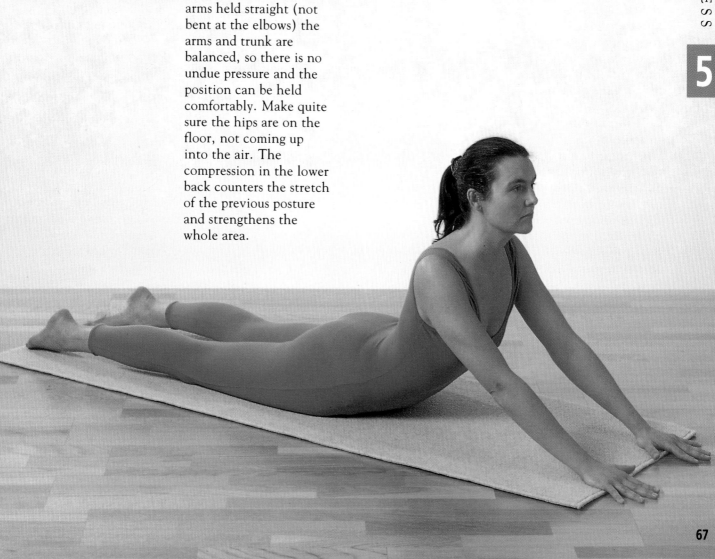

CANDLE MEDITATION

The first requirement of meditation is the power to concentrate – darana in Sanscrit. The realization of this helps you to understand how important meditation is, for everyone knows the value of concentration. The object is to direct the mind to dwell exclusively on one subject. At school children are urged to concentrate and from then on people realize how important concentration is in order to achieve their goals. Yet, in everyday life, we are seldom taught how to concentrate. Meditation, therefore, offering techniques of concentration, is a valuable aid to all aspects of life, from carrying out mundane daily activities to finding a deep peace of mind.

Meditating on a lit candle is a very old practice. It is gentle and calming. It is also a comparatively easy introduction to the art of concentration. Sit erect on the floor or in a chair, having placed the candle a short distance in front of you where you can see it clearly. Gaze steadily at the candle flame for two or three minutes, noting first of all its outline – how steady it is, how it flickers – and then the colours in the flame. Now cover your eyes with your palms and

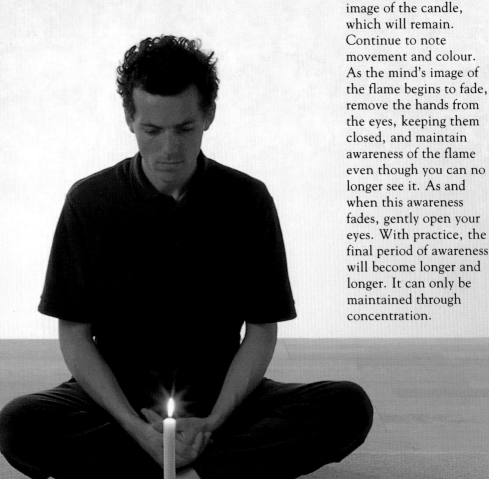

continue to gaze on the image of the candle, which will remain. Continue to note movement and colour. As the mind's image of the flame begins to fade, remove the hands from the eyes, keeping them closed, and maintain awareness of the flame even though you can no longer see it. As and when this awareness fades, gently open your eyes. With practice, the final period of awareness will become longer and longer. It can only be maintained through concentration.

5

USING SOUND

The combination of sound and vision can provide a deep basis for concentration, as we have already seen through the "Hamsa" meditation (see pages 52–53). It has been an Eastern concept for thousands of years that the sound of "Om" (Au-uu-m) is the most sacred of all sounds. It is still chanted daily and, it is claimed, this was the basis of the chant "Amen", used at the end of prayers, hymns and psalms in Christian services.

In the seventeenth century, the astronomer Johannes Kepler declared that each planet had a "song" and he wrote down the individual notations. A few years ago, a professor of music and a professor of geology in America took Kepler's laws and notations and applied them to the motions of the planets. This was fed into a computer connected to a music synthesizer. The result was a "song" of the planets – just as Kepler had argued! If planets in motion must project sound, clearly the sum total of all the objects in motion throughout the universe will also provide a sound. One day we may be able to record this, and no doubt, it will be found to be "Om" – the sound of the universe.

PRACTICE MAKES PERFECT

As with other forms of practice, the more often you perform this, the longer the periods of total concentration you can achieve. You will find the vibration of this amazing sound brings a feeling of harmony that stays with you.

Again, sitting correctly, with the eyes closed, first pay attention to the calm and peaceful rhythm of your breath. After a minute or two, repeat the sound Om (Au-uu-m) to yourself each time you breathe out. Get swept up in the sound, filling your mind, your body, the room . . . everything with it. If your concentration slips, pay attention to your breath and, after a minute or two, open your eyes.

CONTINUING THE PROGRAMME

As you progress, so you grasp the principles more clearly. Yoga is never a matter of learning by rote: it involves getting more and more absorbed in the process so that your individual requirements become apparent. All the different facets are still involved: breathing, postures, relaxation, visualization, meditation – for all are interlinked. Yoga can never be reduced merely to sequences of exercises or techniques. On the other hand, how you blend the elements together will be a matter of personal choice, based on internal awareness.

Before starting your daily programme, sit quietly for a few minutes, clear your mind as fully as possible and, slowly but surely, your needs will become apparent.

5

POSTURES
You are now concerned with development, but this takes place in various ways. Sometimes the new form of a posture will outdate previous performance, in other cases the change is complementary.

Both forms of the Spinal Twist are valuable. Although the earlier one is easier to perform, it provides a really effective twist. The advanced version provides a little more of a challenge, especially if both cheeks of the buttocks are firmly on the ground.

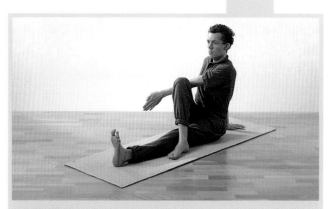

SPINAL TWIST   **Page 25**

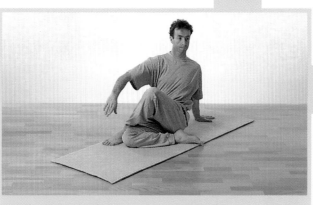

SPINAL TWIST (LEGS BENT)   **Page 65**

The Choking pose is a variation of the Plough. Although the advantages of each have been mentioned, as you progress you will understand for yourself what the posture is achieving – or failing to achieve – by listening to your body. This will enhance life in many ways.

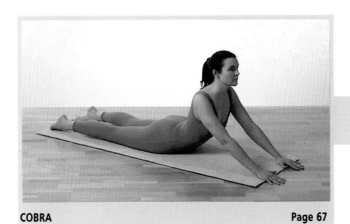

COBRA   **Page 67**

MEDITATION

Meditation benefits you most from being performed every day at the same time and, if possible, in the same place. This is because the brain is happy with reflex patterns; body and brain come to accept it and achieving mental calmness becomes easier. If this is difficult or impossible, just accept that the process will take a little longer. There are many ways in which you can meditate. It is important to find a middle way between experimentation and a jumble of techniques. Proceed quietly and cautiously.

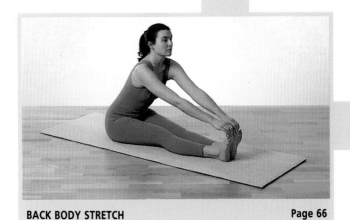

BACK BODY STRETCH   **Page 66**

Your progress with the Back Body Stretch and the Cobra is a more complete achievement. By practising steadily and correctly, with the right mental approach, the body eases itself more and more into a truly effective position.

5

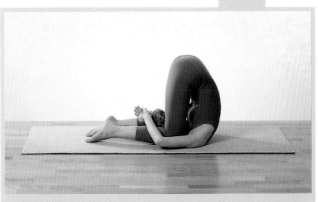

CHOKING POSE   **Page 63**

BREATHING

All aspects of breathing have a role in your regular programme. However, enhancing the natural process and practising the specific *asana* and *pranayama* techniques should also be integrated into daily life. Correct practice will enable you to "top up" your energy and ensure it flows smoothly. A *pranayama* such as the Black Bee will provide a mental stimulus and can be used whenever you have a few minutes alone.

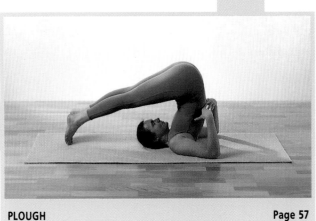

PLOUGH   **Page 57**

MONTH ACTIVE CREATIVITY

6

SIX

AIMS FOR THE MONTH

There is no time when mind and body are not working together, with the brain acting as the go-between. Nobody knows the degree to which we create our own reality, but there are, for example, authenticated cases of stigmata – people actually producing bleeding wounds on their hands and feet by identifying totally in the mind with the Crucifixion. We know that the link between mind and body can be harmful, but we often fail to realize that a strong positive mind/body link can be as beneficial as a negative one can be harmful.

- -

FEELING THE FLOW

Einstein demonstrated that matter equals energy; without energy there is no existence. Energy is a flow – there may be whirls, eddies, torrents, quiet little trickles, but in every aspect it must flow. To be out of ease means a lack of, or obstruction to, the flow of energy: literally, dis-ease.

- -

1 Sitting erect, with the eyes closed, breathe slowly and calmly and, as you breathe in, be aware of the energy rising to the very top of your head.

2 As you breathe out, sense this energy flowing down through every part of the body, right to the fingers and the toes.

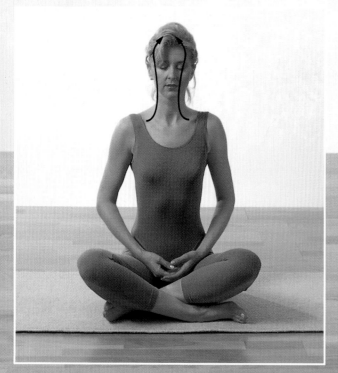
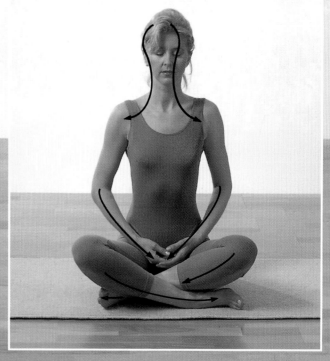

The section on visualization has already outlined the process of creating an effective flow of energy. Carefully monitored tests have shown practitioners changing their body temperature (sometimes in specifically chosen parts of the body), reducing their blood pressure and even controlling the beat of the heart. With practice we can all change aspects of our functioning for the better.

· · · · · · · · · · · · · · · ·

Use the visualization of the flow of energy to tone your whole being, enhancing body function and stimulating mental activity. The sitting position is ideal, either on the floor or in a chair. Keep the back erect but not stiff; link the hands.

Golden mist

With the eyes closed, allow yourself to pay attention to the breath: it should be quite slow and above all rhythmical. Become aware of the in-breath by feeling the cool flow of the air on the nostrils. Create the impression that the air is a golden mist, sun-like in nature.

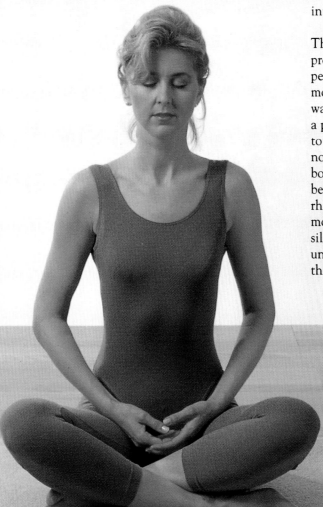

As you breathe in, this golden mist links with the warmth of your body and rises to the top of your head. As you breathe out, it flows right down through every part of the body into the fingers and toes.

The object of this process is, through calm persistence, to identify more and more with this warm, golden flow; to be a part of its rise and fall; to feel it move into every nook and cranny of the body. Your whole being becomes one harmonious rhythm: a glorious ballet movement, a wave of silk in the breeze, an undulation of water in the ocean.

6

INSTANT RELAXATION

It is so easy to let things seize you up that you tend to think it is inevitable, and that you can do nothing about it. Many major problems start with minor ones that go uncorrected and just grow, almost undetected.

Right at the start, the need for stretching, releasing the neck and shoulders and simply swinging energy into the body were emphasized. All these quite simple things need to become a part of life, used when the body signals tension or lack of energy.

Other equally simple actions are shown here in an office setting, but they could be performed equally well in the home or elsewhere.

1 Many activities cramp the body, slow circulation and limit muscle function. To counteract this, work the shoulders and the back for a minute or so, then take the hands and link the fingers as you place them on the back of the head, elbows out.

2 Take a deep breath in and, as you breathe out, press the head down, bringing the chin against the neck and the elbows closer together. Feel the strong stretch on the back of the neck. Hold the position until you feel the need to breathe in again and then release. Repeat at least three times.

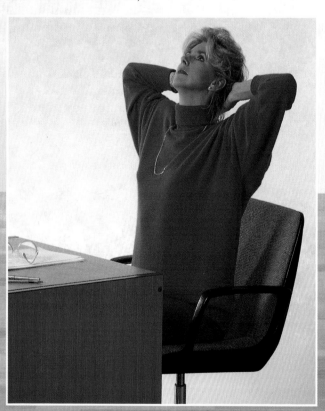

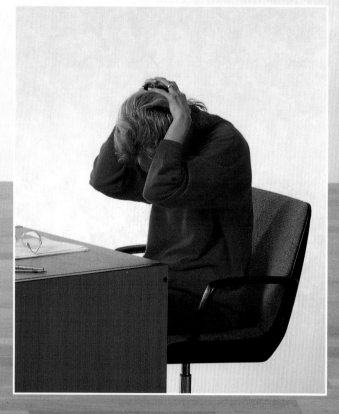

Much of our time at work is spent with back and shoulders hunched. This is uncomfortable in the short term and can become serious in time. Apart from the sitting stretch, also perform the standing one already shown (see page 22), even if it is not practical to carry out the whole sequence.

(see page 22)

· ·

It is not always practical to get up and move about; an effective stretch can be carried out while seated in a chair. Link the fingers, letting hands lie on the lap. Breathe in, stretch the arms into the air, turning the hands so that the palms are uppermost. Get the arms level with the ears and straighten them, still stretching up. Hold until the impulse comes to breathe out and then come slowly down. This also should be repeated at least three times.

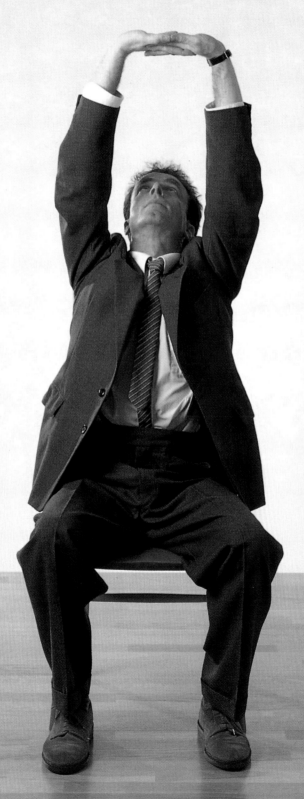

ENCOURAGING BENEFICIAL REFLEXES

The biggest problem with simple but important stretches is remembering to do them! The more stiff, irked and dejected we get, the less likely we are to do anything about it. That is one of the values of a book like this. Keep it where you will look at it regularly. Leaf through the pages day-by-day and take note of the reminders. After a while a pattern of reflexes becomes established, and you start to reap benefits.

INSTANT RELAXATION

6

BODY AND MIND

Using the body to quieten the mind and enhance inner peace, together with the capacity to act, is a concept little understood in the West. Using the body is considered to be a physical process only and using the mind is not really understood at all. If these two central aspects of life are brought together, your whole outlook changes. You come to realize there is a new dimension to living. The examples given in this book are only "for instances". The one below will probably be something of a surprise, because it is a variation on a standard form of stretching.

1 Standing with the legs just a little apart, breathe out and as you breathe in stretch the arms out to the side and over the head. Lift high.

2 Then start stretching up with the right arm, pulling up the whole of the right side.

3 Alternate with the left arm and, after at least a dozen times with each arm, have a final strong stretch up with both arms. Bring the arms down on an out-breath. While performing the stretch fill yourself with a feeling of rejoicing. Liberate the whole body with a joyous feeling.

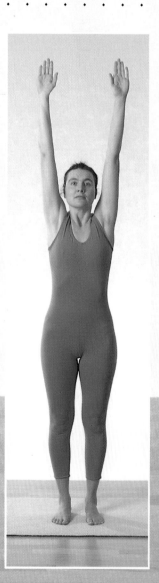
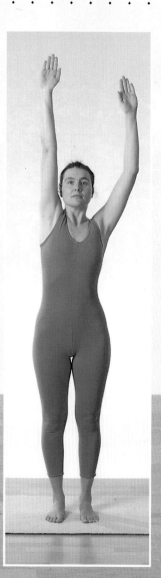
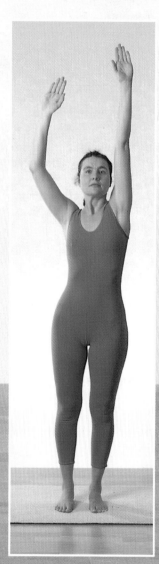

Yoga is a process of self-realization. While this book aims to provide information and hints on how to proceed, you, the reader, are your own most valuable teacher. Any book can do no more than provide a few examples, for the subject is immense. Once you have grasped the concept that the body functions better when a calm, controlled mind lets it do so, you can then apply the idea to a whole variety of postures.

The Simple Tree.
Mental and physical balance go together, something which is not fully realized. Prayer in India is often combined with physical movements. Today you still see devotees standing on the banks of the Ganges, balanced on one leg, with the hands in the *namaste* (prayer position) on the chest. Their eyes are closed and they are reciting a prayer.

Place one foot on the opposite knee, letting the knee of the bent leg fall outwards. Place the hands together on the chest and close the eyes. Repeat to yourself a thought or saying you find helpful, or say a prayer. The length of time you can hold this will increase with practice. Repeat the process with the other leg.

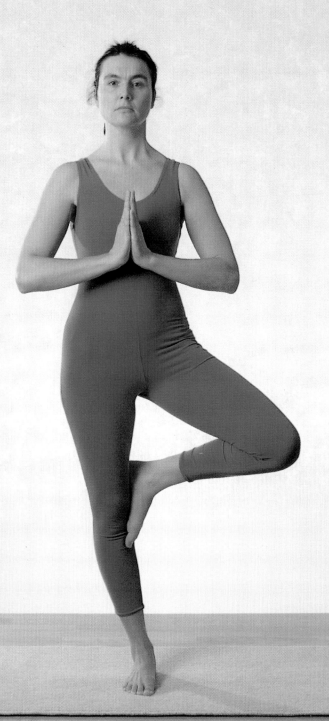

BODY AND MIND

6

CONTINUING THE PROGRAMME

Developing a consistent approach to life is of primary importance. Naturally, we all experience many different moods; these will arise for a variety of reasons. Quite apart from events, our outlook is also influenced by fluctuations in our flow of energy and a hundred-and-one other internal causes. But behind all these factors lies the steady process we call consciousness and this enables us to bring about beneficial changes when everyday factors make us dispirited, angry, lethargic or frustrated.

This is why the daily programme should never be reduced to a series of exercises. True physical benefit stems from true mental benefit and this is an integration of the different factors that make up life.

6

No-one can see the processes upon which life is based but, although invisible, these life forces *flow*. If we are "open" mentally and physically that flow enhances our life. Tensions and strains, both in mind and body, block the flow, with highly damaging results.

VISUALIZATION
Visualizing these invisible forces as a golden mist, breathing slowly and calmly, sitting quietly and naturally, enhances all aspects of life. It is combined with postures and should also be carried out regularly on its own.

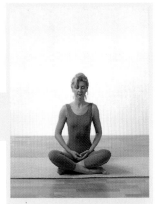

Page 72

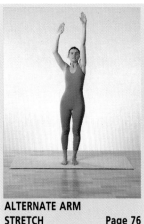

ALTERNATE ARM STRETCH   **Page 76**

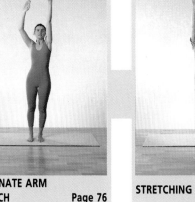

STRETCHING   **Page 22**

POSTURES
Even simple stretching movements need to be holistic. You can now add the alternate arm stretch to the original sequence. Feel the movements as an expression of vitality.

The Tree and the Mountain have much in common. Steadiness of balance on one leg, with the hands in the prayer position, directs your attention upwards. Similarly, the Mountain stretch is an expression of exultation, linking earth and the heavens.

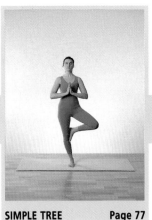

SIMPLE TREE   **Page 77**

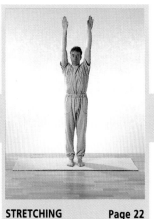

MOUNTAIN BREATH   **Page 54**

Moving from the Pose of Tranquility, which is largely in the air, into the Plough, which gives the feeling of being grounded, involves somewhat varying moods.

The following two poses always go together. It is useful to perform the simple head and neck exercises first and ensure the shoulders are always flexible.

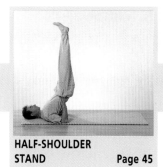

HALF-SHOULDER STAND Page 45

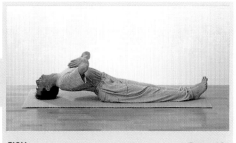

FISH Page 46

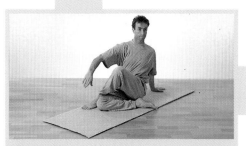

SPINAL TWIST (LEGS BENT) Page 65

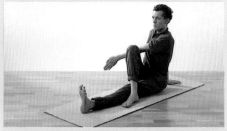

SPINAL TWIST Page 25

The following two poses also go together. Listen to your body: it will quickly show you any ways in which you are unbalanced as well as the ways in which it is being benefited.

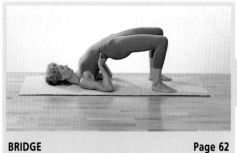

BRIDGE Page 62

Performing the two versions of the Spinal Twist provides a more complete "work out" and helps you to become aware of the effect of similar yet different bodily movements.

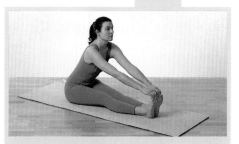

BACK BODY STRETCH Page 66

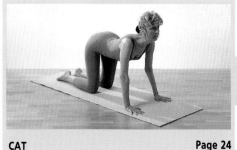

CAT Page 24

The flexibility of the back induced by the Cat is a good preliminary to the Bridge.

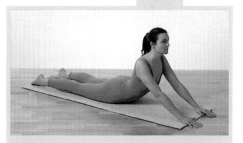

COBRA Page 67

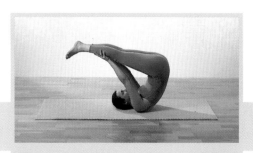

POSE OF TRANQUILITY Page 56

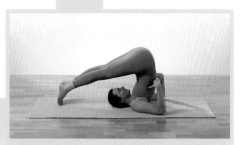

PLOUGH Page 57

MEDITATION
Meditation is the king of practices because it takes you beyond the body. This does not mean ignoring the body, but accepting it, while realizing there is something much deeper.

6

THE YOGA DAY

Yoga offers a singularly comprehensive approach to life: profound thoughts about existence and the universe on one hand, and how to avoid the pitfalls that generate both unhappiness and illness on the other. As you know, water dripping constantly can make a hole in a stone. Our inability to react effectively to small challenges creates a mental and physical build-up which can be very damaging. Try to counteract this by planning your days more effectively.

EARLY MORNING

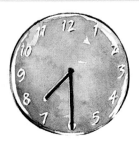

Remember the importance of opening up the breath, de-tensing and stretching. Setting a standard for the day with a thought or a short reading can be of immense benefit. Build up concentration, too, by doing chores, such as washing, cleaning your teeth, brushing your hair, with care. Doing one thing and thinking of another leads to confusion.

MID·MORNING

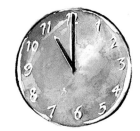

Remember that you can concentrate for relatively short periods – effectively for about an hour. Take regular short breaks. A few minutes' relief will actually heighten your capacity to understand and remember. Saying, "I'm too busy to stop" will usually end in slipshod results. All too often over-concentration and physical tension go together. Even small movements like working the shoulders and the neck can make a big difference. Above all, pay attention to the need for quiet natural breathing.

LUNCHTIME

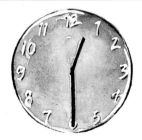

Digestion is a complex process. Snatching a snack can be harmful and slouching over a meal can turn the digestive process into a torture. Getting into the habit of eating carefully will pay dividends. The busy or slapdash person will ruin a day by sloppy eating habits.

AFTERNOON

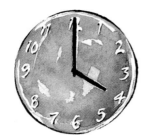

The afternoon can be quite a dangerous time! Digestion is a slow process, requiring an effective flow of blood in the abdominal area. Good erect posture will help health and happiness, by allowing the system to function well. Mental and physical capacity is generally lowered for a while. A short rest, a walk or some other sensible way of letting the body function quietly can be immensely beneficial. Millions of people these days work in front of computers and other apparatus and all these things tend to affect posture, lower energy levels and interfere with the effective working of the muscles. Good posture, calm breathing and regular short breaks are essential.

EARLY EVENING

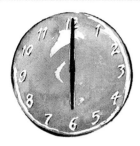

For very many people, the early evening is a transition period, moving from work into evening activities. This is one of the best times to combine a wash, bath or shower with at least a short session of yoga *asanas,* followed by relaxation and awareness of breathing. With such a break, one feels a "new person". Energy is topped up and the evening becomes far more enjoyable.

BEDTIME

Too many people allow the day to build up mental and physical tensions and then jump straight into bed, only to wonder why they do not sleep properly. Preparing for bed requires getting the mind into a relaxed state, so that sleep can follow naturally. Some gentle, but effective, stretching helps to start this process and a few minutes of calm, rhythmical breathing will underline the process. It is good, also, to remind oneself that the capacity to deal with matters on the following day will depend, at least in part, on a good night's sleep. In bed, listen to the breath and liken it to the wavelets of a calm sea breaking on the shore.

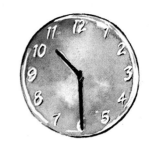

Many people may feel that such simple, everyday matters cannot be linked with yoga, but an examination of the traditional writings reveals that yogis have always understood that the small points of life are closely linked to the big issues. If we establish a simple but effective pattern to see us through each day, then the major activities and challenges will be dealt with much more effectively.

ABOUT ENERGY

AIMS FOR THE MONTH

The human body is a mass of electro-magnetic fields, in an electro-magnetic world, which is part of an electro-magnetic universe. Some of the body's electric energy is generated by the pumping of the heart, but "no man is an island" and we share this wonderful mixture of waves, vibrations, electro-magnetism and gases, which is termed the air or the atmosphere. The term used for it in yoga is prana, which can be translated as "life force". In this month, while keeping up the practice to date, devote your main attention to this force.

. . . .

THE PSYCHOLOGY OF THE BREATH

Physical and mental stresses and strains will always affect the natural flow of breath, so we will never reach a stage in which we can afford to ignore the day-by-day process.

. . . .

1 Breath is intimately bound up with every aspect of life. To breathe in, you have to draw the air into the lungs. If you are unhappy, your in-breath is very poor.

2 In the normal out-breath the air is simply allowed to flow out, a relaxed and peaceful movement. A tense person finds breathing out very difficult.

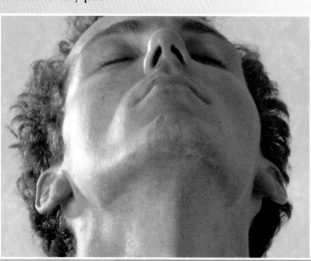

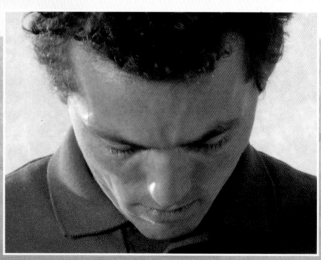

ENERGY CENTRES

Electro-magnetically based energy flows through the body and corresponds with the Chinese concept of acupuncture, now recognized in the West and used by many doctors. The yoga concept is that the body has a series of energy centres, known as *chakras*, (*Chakra* means a wheel or vortex.) These are situated parallel with the spine. While yet insufficiently researched, the evidence for the existence of these centres is growing.

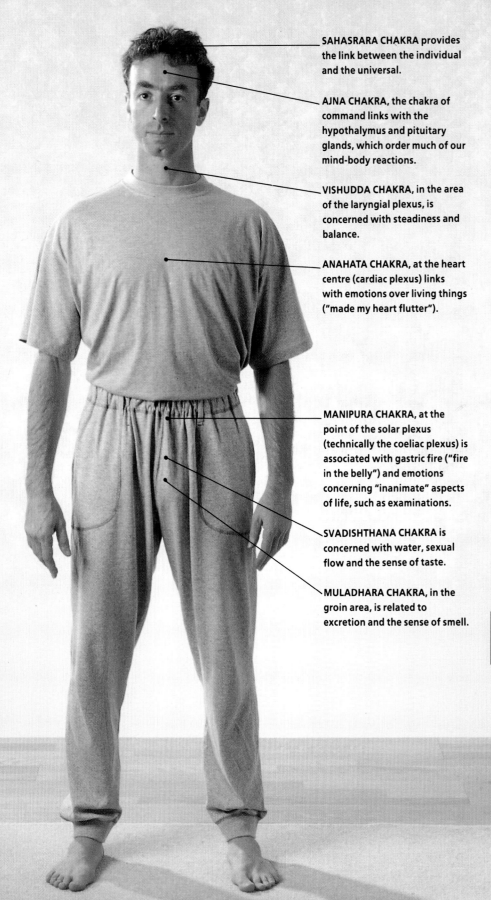

SAHASRARA CHAKRA provides the link between the individual and the universal.

AJNA CHAKRA, the chakra of command links with the hypothalymus and pituitary glands, which order much of our mind-body reactions.

VISHUDDA CHAKRA, in the area of the laryngial plexus, is concerned with steadiness and balance.

ANAHATA CHAKRA, at the heart centre (cardiac plexus) links with emotions over living things ("made my heart flutter").

MANIPURA CHAKRA, at the point of the solar plexus (technically the coeliac plexus) is associated with gastric fire ("fire in the belly") and emotions concerning "inanimate" aspects of life, such as examinations.

SVADISHTHANA CHAKRA is concerned with water, sexual flow and the sense of taste.

MULADHARA CHAKRA, in the groin area, is related to excretion and the sense of smell.

THE ALTERNATE NOSTRIL BREATH

A series of special yoga breathing techniques
go by the Sanscrit name of pranayama.
Literally this means "interruption of breath".
It involves taking control of breathing to
achieve particular purposes. For most of the
time we breathe predominantly through one
nostril or the other. Only for about 20 per
cent of the time do we breathe equally through
both nostrils. Breathing corresponds with the
positive and negative aspects in electrical
terms. The Alternate Nostril Breath ensures
effective functioning of each nostril and assists
in the balance of energy. It is one of the oldest
pranayama techniques.

1 Bring up the right
hand and close the
right nostril with the
thumb; bend down the
first and second fingers
and place the third finger
by the left nostril.
Breathe in, to a count of
four, keeping the right
nostril closed.

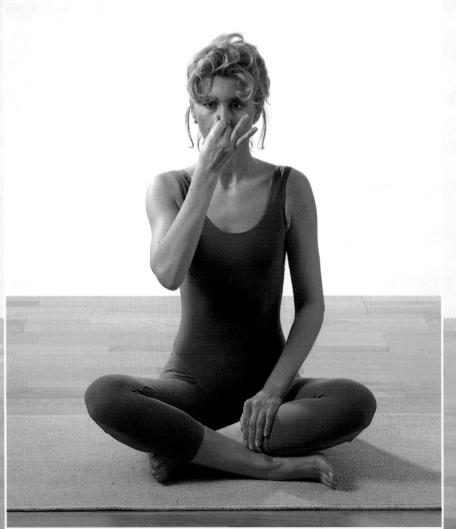

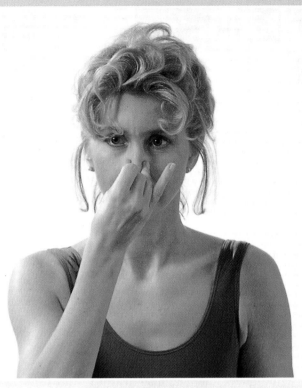

2 Close the left nostril with the third finger and retain the breath for a count of 16.

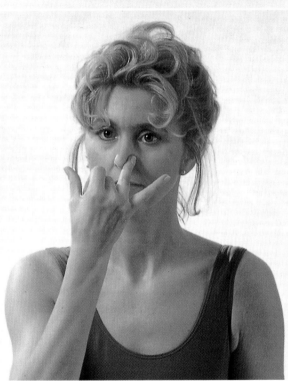

3 Take the thumb away from the right nostril and breathe slowly out to a count of eight. Then reverse the process, breathing in through the right nostril and, after retaining, out through the left. This completes one round. Start with four or five rounds; build up until you can do at least a dozen rounds comfortably.

Another valuable *pranayama* is called the Black Bee. For this, sitting erect, you breathe deeply in and briefly retain the breath. Then very slowly breathe out through the open mouth, making the sound of "ung" – as in "gung". This will sound remarkably similar to the buzzing of the bee, setting up a valuable vibration through the whole body. Repeat at least three times.

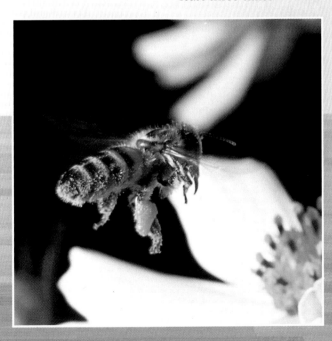

THE BELLOWS BREATH

Long ago humans discovered that blowing on a fire caused it to blaze up. For many years they must have been content to use the muscles of their own trunks to achieve this effect. Then, based on their physiological experience, they created the bellows. This directs a strong and beneficial force: the yoga *pranayama* called the Bellows Breath uses that force within the human framework to tone up the system.

Energizing the body

Natural breathing involves tensing the muscles to draw air into the lungs (usually an automatic process) and then releasing them to let the air flow out again. A bellows reverses this process: it expels the air forcefully and then allows it to flow passively in again. Curiously enough, this is akin to the process by which we laugh heartily. A "belly laugh" consists of ejecting the air on the "Ha" sound and then letting it flow back in. The whole process is a fast one, resulting in the body being energized. Not only is oxygen pumped vigorously into the bloodstream, the diaphragm also pumps sharply, stimulating the body's electro-magnetic flow. This is why laughter has been discovered to be a first-class therapy, so much so that some American hospitals now employ clowns and comics to make the patients laugh.

Stimulating the brain

Not only is the body stimulated beneficially in this way, the brain is helped too. We tend not to realize that the brain has a mobile structure, it pulsates. This pulsation is a direct stimulation of its functions and is affected by the breath. Hearty laughter – or the performance of the yoga Bellows Breath – speeds up the breathing process greatly and this, in turn, stimulates the mental pulsation. Another breathing process akin to the Bellows Breath is called the Shining Head. The first stimulates the whole body, the latter specifically works on the head and the brain.

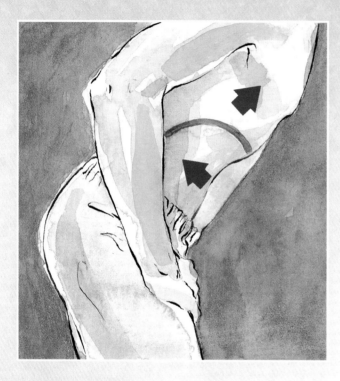

The Bellows Breath.
This can be performed either sitting or standing. While the back should be erect, it can be tilted forward and the hands placed on the thighs to allow free play to the muscles. Having breathed in, the breath should be ejected sharply through the nostrils, the abdominal muscles contracted to enforce the process. Then the air is allowed to flow back in to the lungs. Having practised the movements, you can then speed up the process so the breathing becomes very rapid. The sound of the air through the nose on the out-breath will resemble a bellows sound. Somewhere between 10 and 20 such breaths form one round. This should be followed by a slow deep breath in, which is retained for some seconds and then slowly exhaled. Two or three rounds will be quite sufficient, even when one is proficient.

The Shining Head.
This is performed similarly, but whereas in the Bellows Breath the abdomen is controlled on the in-breath, in the Shining Head it is allowed to expand. As a result, on the sharp out-breath the force is more precisely directed upwards. The many benefits of these processes are obvious, but, as with yoga *asanas*, the important thing is to concentrate on the mental benefits, noticing the brain clarity that arises. Circulation, lung function and the whole neuro-muscular system will all benefit.

PRACTISING PRANAYAMA

Pranayama can be practised in complete sessions, but, if you are integrating yoga into your daily life it is important to understand the particular benefits that each technique provides and to use them accordingly.

Remember, yoga gives you the opportunity of bringing life under your own control to a remarkable degree. Instead of just complaining, combat physical symptoms appropriately.

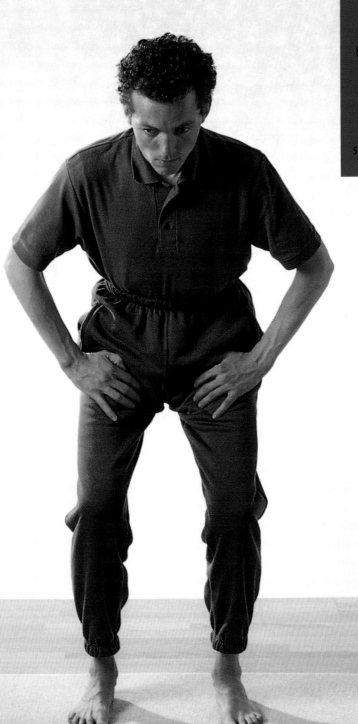

THE BELLOWS BREATH

7

THE RABBIT

This is a relatively recent yoga practice and
is a good way of exercising the three lobe
areas of the lungs. It gets its name from the
fact that the first two parts resemble a rabbit
squatting and sitting up. The third section,
sometimes called the Hare, may possibly be
thought to resemble a mad, March hare. The
first movement opens the abdominal area,
the second the thoracic (rib-cage) area and
the third the clavicular (upper trunk) area.

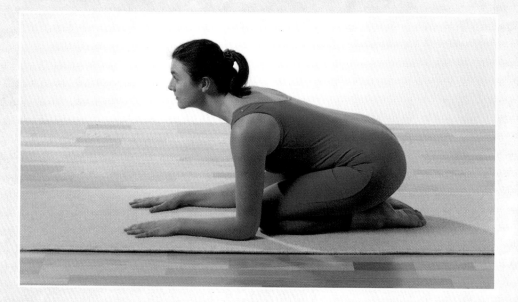

1 Sit back on the
heels, with the
forearms on the floor in
front of the legs, palms
downwards. Look ahead
of you. As you breathe
out, quite slowly
contract the abdominal
muscles, pulling away
from the thighs.
Breathing in, allow
the abdomen to
expand, pressing against
the thighs. Repeat
several times.

2 Now sit up on the
heels, hands palms
down just ahead of the
knees. Again look
ahead. Breathing out
again, contract the
abdominal muscles. This
time, on the in-breath
the bottom ribs only
will expand. Repeat
several times.

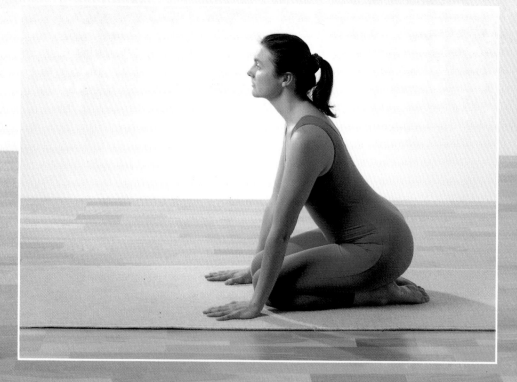

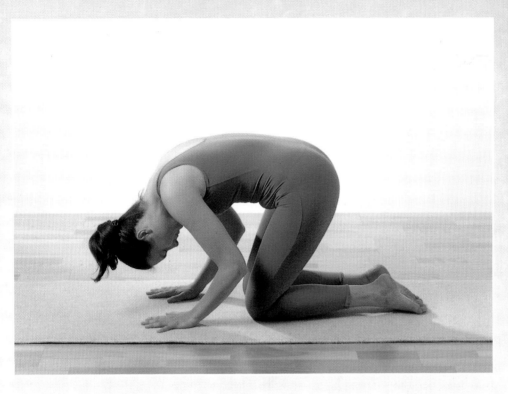

Using the lungs effectively and keeping them free from congestion, is of great importance. Shallow breathing can lead to the lungs holding stagnant air and the passages becoming blocked. Freeing the passageways keeps the lung tissue in a good state and is vital for effective oxygenation of the blood.

3 Bring the hands a little further forward, breathe in and, as you breathe out, bring the crown of the head on to the floor.

4 When the head is firmly on the floor, swing the body forward as you breathe in and swing it back as you breathe out. After several rounds come slowly up on an in-breath.

THE RABBIT

7

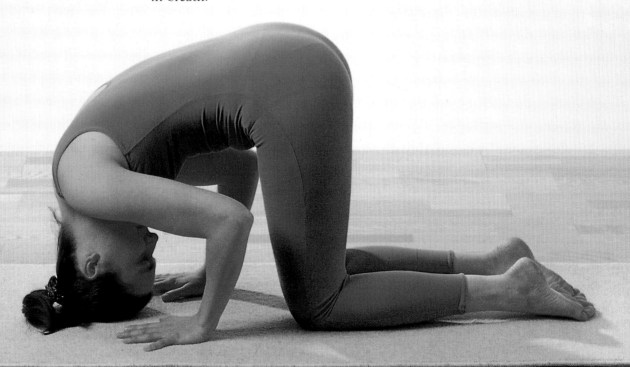

RETAINING THE BREATH

Respiration is an automatic process and we are born with reflexes that enable us to adapt the breath to the needs of the moment. But we also have voluntary, or conscious, control of breathing, so that when things go wrong we have the ability to put them right.

. . . .

By means of quiet intuition and experimentation, yogis realized a long time ago that the control of breathing involves not only inhalation and exhalation, but also the way in which the breath is retained. They called the stopping of the breath, *kumbhaka*, and they pointed out that we have the capacity to stop our breathing for a short while after inhaling and after exhaling. They also pointed out that breathing could be brought to a stop at any time and this they regarded as the most important attribute. A central reason for stopping the breath is its effect on the brain and the mind.

When something happens suddenly, causing the necessity of making an instant decision, you stop breathing immediately. If you are driving your car and someone steps out into the road in front of you, you hold your breath without a fraction of a delay. This is because this concentrates the mind totally for a short period while you brake, swerve or take any other action. Even a delay of a second or so could be fatal.

This instant *kumbhaka* concentrates the mind. Retaining the breath after inhalation helps sedate the mind, putting it into a state of calmness, which enhances the process of meditation.

. . . .

Sit either on the floor or on a chair in a correct position and close the eyes. Breathe slowly and naturally for a minute or two. Take a deep breath in and drop the head so the chin is pressing against the chest. Let the trunk muscles relax so you feel you are sitting on a cushion of air. Keep the breath in and let your mind dwell on a sense of stillness. Do not worry about the breath, just bathe in this state of total non-action. After a while you will feel the need to breathe again becoming strong. Raise the head, lift the trunk and *gently* breathe out. Let the breathing adjust itself naturally.

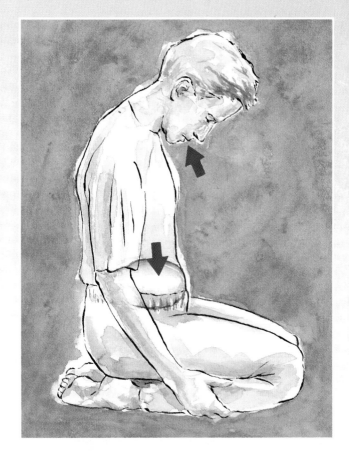

BREATH AND BALANCE

Remember that the words for breathing in and out are "inspire" and "expire". Here lies the fundamental balance of existence. The trinity of being is seen in the breath: creation, with the in-breath; preservation, as the breath is retained and, although in one sense breathing out signifies destruction, this is in fact only the process of change. From the breath you rejoice in life and embrace change.

7

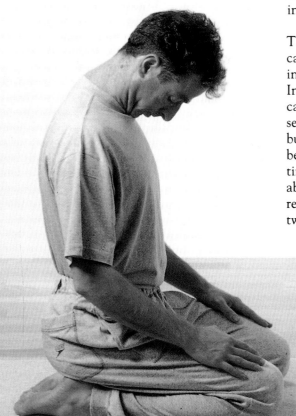

Repeat two or three times, but always take some stabilizing breaths in between.

The length of time you can hold the breath will increase with practice. In the early stages you can check against the second hand of a watch, but give this up as you become more adept. In time you are likely to be able to manage a retention in excess of two minutes.

Remember, this is not a test of endurance but a process taking you towards greater control of body and mind.

Clearly those with heart conditions, or suffering from hypertension, will not attempt this.

CONTINUING THE PROGRAMME

Conscious concern about the breath involves three distinct approaches. The first is to ensure that the breath is functioning naturally, on the one hand pumping energy through the body and brain, on the other allowing the organism to relax and let go. The multitude of problems, physical and mental, that are endemic in our civilization, disrupt natural breathing patterns.

A second approach is to use the breath in conjunction with movement. In cases such as the Mountain, these become breathing asanas.

The third approach is controlling the breath to produce specific benefits. This we call pranayama.

BREATHING
Breath is energy and the diaphragm is the pump involved: using it ensures full use of the lungs and the flow of the body's electro-magnetic force. Becoming aware of the rhythmical movement of the bottom ribs, while the rest of the trunk remains still, is most important.

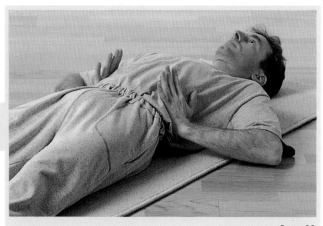

Page 33

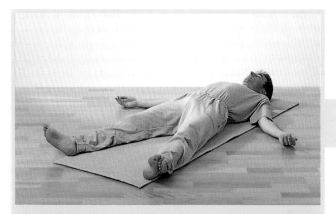

RELAXATION   Page 31

When you relax, the pumping action is greatly reduced. As a result of the relaxation, the abdomen will rise gently on the in-breath and fall slowly on the exhalation. It is important to stay aware of this.

If you want to keep muscles in tone for strong physical or sporting activities, the strong breathing postures, such as the Mountain, are invaluable, because they enhance the electrical flow along the nervous system and build up muscle tone.

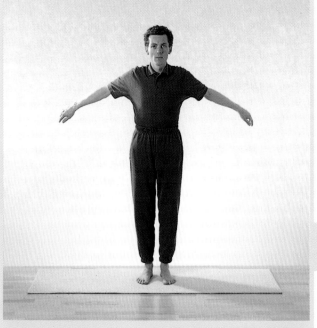

MOUNTAIN BREATH   Page 54

7

POSTURES

It is easy to counsel perfection, but we are not living in a perfect world. There will be days when it does not seem possible to spend more than, say, ten minutes on postures. Don't think it is not worth it – just concentrate on the four basic movements of the trunk.

These basic movements – stretching forwards, backwards, twisting and bending sideways – with an opening stretch and a short final relaxation, will provide a mini-session of considerable value. The following poses are just one possible combination; you can develop your own mini-session.

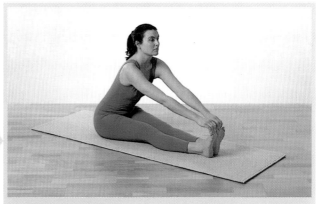

BACK BODY STRETCH   Page 66

A *pranayama* technique such as the Bee is very helpful, because it combines control of the breath with a strong vibratory sound. It becomes fascinating to feel how the body responds to the sound and this helps us to understand – and wish to explore – the relationship between vibration, resonance and health.

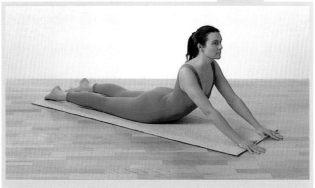

COBRA   Page 67

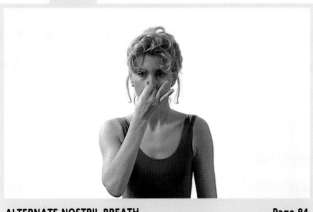

ALTERNATE NOSTRIL BREATH   Page 84

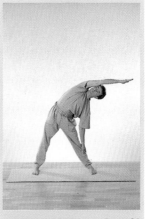

SIDEWAYS BEND   Page 64

Move into *pranayama* techniques with caution. The Alternate Nostril Breath is really the basis of such techniques, because it balances the internal energy system, providing a central role in what is termed homeostasis. However, it should be built up slowly. Both the number of rounds and the lengths of individual components of the breath – in, hold, out – should be increased over a reasonable period. Do not try to do too much, too soon.

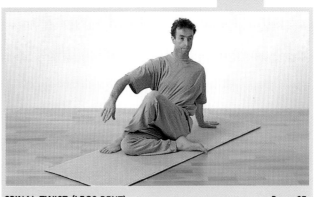

SPINAL TWIST (LEGS BENT)   Page 65

BRAIN CONTROL

AIMS FOR THE MONTH

Control of physical actions begins in infancy. At the same time, babies start to distinguish sounds and associate them with verbal and pictorial images. As the physical body increasingly comes under control, so the role of the mind is enhanced. Gradually, self-awareness – the link between self and the surrounding world – becomes central to our lives. Yet people all too easily assume that they cannot control their thoughts, although learning to control the brain and to use the mind constructively is the greatest adventure in life. This month the focus is on linking such control with all aspects of life.

· ·

COOLNESS AND CREATIVITY

For thousands of years, yoga teachings have insisted that human beings have one aspect of energy or force on one side of the body and a different one on the other, the two interlinking to provide a balanced life. The force on the left side, called Ida, is related to the coolness of the moon and is the calculating aspect of life. That on the right, Pingala, relates to the warmth of the sun and the process of creativity.

· · · · · · · · · · · · · ·

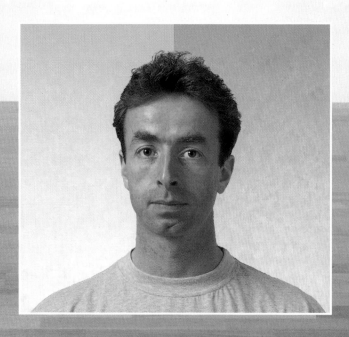

In recent years, neuro-scientists have established that the left hemisphere of the brain is associated with verbal activity and numeracy – the cool, calculating aspects – and the right hemisphere controls our creative processes – in other words, exactly what the yogis had been saying for centuries.

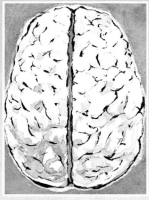

The brain is divided into two hemispheres: the left hemisphere controls the calculating aspects of life, the right controls creativity.

The importance of balance

Life is a question of balance. Tension, or will-power, is necessary but it must be balanced with relaxation, or letting-go. This "letting-go" is based upon the in-and-out flow of the breath, upon which all mental and physical functions are based.

Self-awareness, the basis of consciousness, is an instrument by which life can be both developed and enhanced mentally and physically. If, however, you abrogate control of the brain you abrogate control of life itself; used negatively, self-awareness can become destructive. The choice between creation or destruction lies in our own hands.

Once you are aware, you can use that awareness either positively or negatively. The brain and the body are actually the servants of consciousness.

Creating balance

Bearing in mind the need for balance in all things – sometimes called the middle way – you can review your life and see how far you make use of the cool, logical aspects on the one hand and how far you indulge in creativity in all its forms on the other.

Our present society could well be regarded as left-brain orientated. Once you bring into your life the immense powers of visualization and meditation, and balance tensions with relaxation, you are in a position to contemplate the functions of the brain and to establish the understanding that balance between them is of immense importance. This will, in turn, affect the way you look at many aspects of your life. Beneficial changes then take place, not because you have puzzled about them and calculated them, but because it is part of a natural process.

8

OVERCOMING RESENTMENT

Medical research has shown that a prime cause of ill-health – sometimes even death – is resentment. In overcoming negative emotions you do not deny actual happenings, but move on from them. Visualization can play a major role in helping to achieve this.

1 Sit quietly and imagine that you are with a group of people, sitting in a circle. In front of each of you is a small mound of modelling clay. It is plastic, but has an unpleasant, muddy colour.

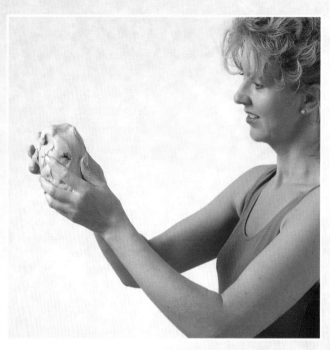

2 Pick up the pile of clay and begin to mould it with your fingers. As you do so, the unpleasant colour reminds you of the resentments you feel about people and events, for such resentments always feel dark and heavy.

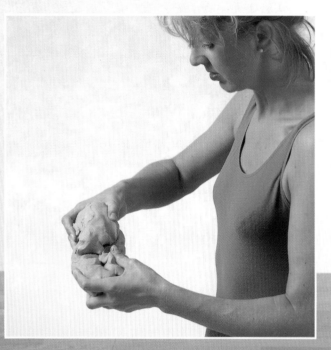

3 Knead your resentments into the clay, to bury them in it. Draw the unpleasant thoughts from your mind and squeeze them into the clay.

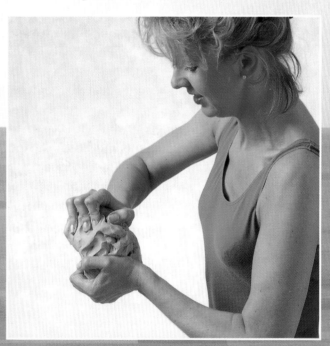

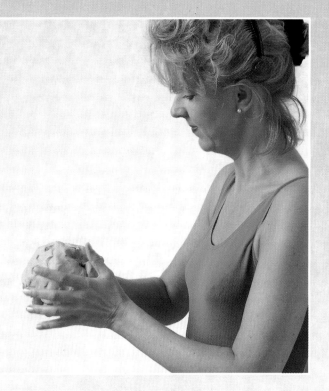

4 Finally you – and all the imaginary people around you – make a single pile of the clay on the floor and you realize it contains all your resentments. Imagine that a man with a barrow comes in, shovels the clay on to the barrow, and takes it away. You then visualize him digging a hole, tipping all the clay into it and replacing the soil. You feel a wonderful sense of lightness as you realize your heavy thoughts have been buried for ever. Now you can move on freely once more.

SUCCESSFUL VISUALIZATION

Visualization is like playing a game: to be successful, it demands your whole concentration. Let the scene and the actions be wholly real to you. Although you do not literally have to see the setting, you create an intense awareness of it. The more completely you join in the concept, the more effective the result will be.

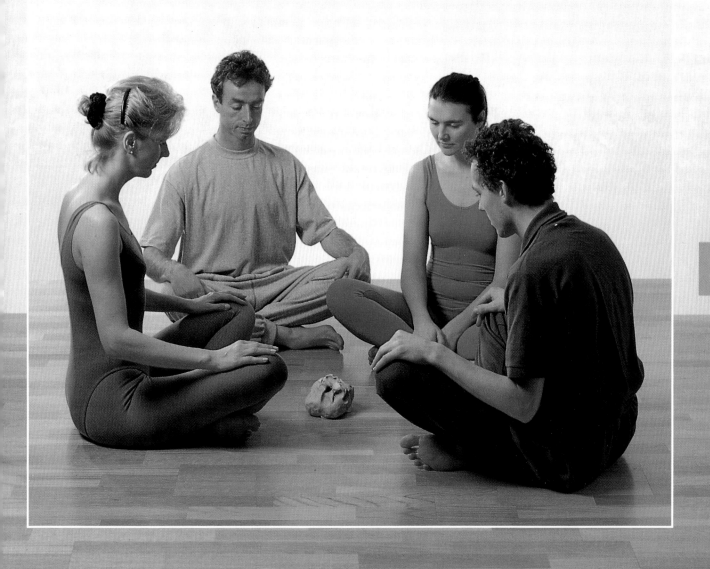

COUNTERING THE SENSES

The messages our senses provide are thought of as "reality". In fact, sensory reaction is determined by circumstances and habit. For example, in a temperate country, where the temperature was 20°C (68°F), a native inhabitant would regard it as a nice, warm day, a visitor newly-arrived from Alaska would find it stiflingly hot, while another from Central Africa would be shivering in the cold. Similar analogies can be provided for the other senses. It is important to realize that the senses are very useful but no-one should be a slave to them.

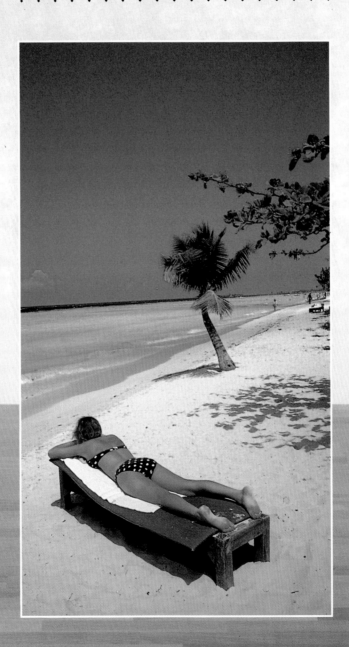

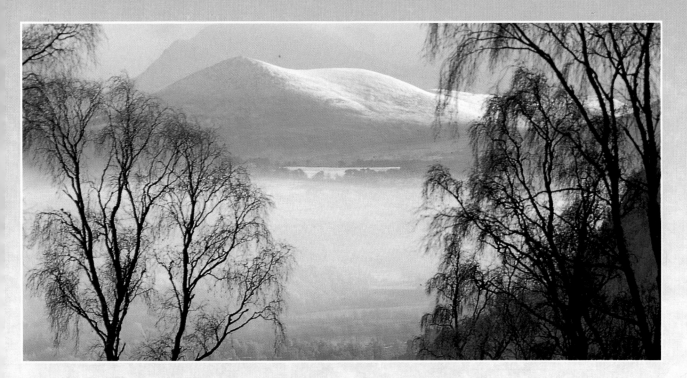

Some people become particularly fond of food, for example. At lunchtime their senses remind them a meal is due. The fact that they are well fed and could defer or do without the meal makes no difference. They become unhappy and fret if food is not to hand. Even if there is a good reason for the meal being delayed, they still worry about its absence. The resulting agitation harms the body. In turn, the body feeds back unhappy signals to the brain and a vicious circle begins. In due course real psychophysical harm ensues. The yoga philosophy develops a spirit of detachment in which the signals of the senses are regarded as useful indicators, but not necessarily as imperative demands. The resulting mental stability, when such a state is achieved, establishes a brain/body harmony that makes for balance, conservation of energy and enhanced well-being.

State of mind and temperature

In Tibet, where it can sometimes be extremely cold, yogis have shown how they can inure themselves to such conditions, maintaining their body heat. A few years ago, Professor Herbert Benson, of Harvard Medical School was able, with the help of the Dalai Lama, to carry out clinical tests on yogis in India. These showed the yogis could select a specific part of the body, such as a finger, and change its temperature by visualization, a process usually described as will-power.

Susceptibility to temperature plays a major role in many people's lives. Although you could adjust the amount of clothing, this is not always possible. Adjusting the state of mind can produce substantial results.

A man living in the Far East found the cold nights very trying and believed he just could not get warm in bed. He consulted a yogi to obtain advice and the yogi told him to visualize a large, glowing ball of golden heat, which came nearer and nearer. He knew that this heat could not singe, burn or hurt him, so he could relax into its rays. He did this every night, and before long his wife moved into another bed, complaining her husband's body was getting too hot!

One effective way of countering a feeling of coolness or cold is to sit correctly, with the eyes closed and recollect a holiday in which you lay on a beach in hot sunshine. If some feeling of cold persists, recall that coming out of the water you have felt a little chilly until the sun has dried your body and again feel the sun at work. If you do this calmly and with assurance, you will be surprised at the result. You can use the same technique, with a different visualization, to counteract feeling overheated. In both cases, the strength of your concentration will make the brain respond to the visualization, rather than the senses.

MIND AND MOVEMENT

The more asanas we perform, the more important it becomes to practise them as an integration of mind-energy-body. Not only does this enhance the performance of the asana itself, it also stimulates the mental processes and will result in an improved quality of life. Every movement can be linked to a mental concept. Once the principles are firmly understood, the visualization can vary, but do not indulge in change for the sake of it. Once you find suitable imagery, it is as well to keep to it, at least most of the time.

The Palm Tree. This is a simple but important posture in which the body is well-stretched above the hips (and legs and hips, too, benefit from the lightening of the load above). It is all too easy to perform this as an unthinking exercise. Resist this temptation.

Stand with the feet 3-4in (8-10cm) apart, toes pointing to the front. Having breathed out, stretch the arms out to the sides and up until you are reaching as high as you can. Retain the breath as you hold the stretch and breathe slowly out as the arms come down. Repeat several times.

Be the tree while you are doing this. Link the arm movements to a light breeze and the final stretch to the tall tree, reaching up to heaven. Feel the sun and the sense of growth.

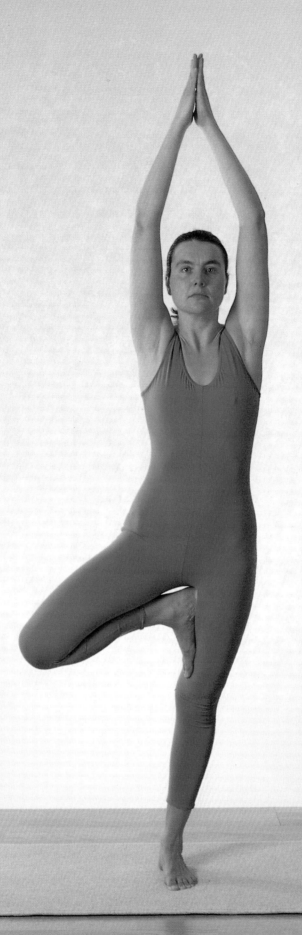

The Tree. You have already performed a relatively simple one-legged posture, noting that it comes from a prayer position. Now you can develop this as an *asana* known as the Tree. Once more the visualization is that you are a tree, but this time you are one with many branches. In your mind's eye see the tree on a still day and then feel you have become that tree.

Bring one leg up with the foot into the groin and let the knee fall back in line with the straight leg. On an in-breath, stretch to the side and up, finally bringing the palms together, maintaining the stretch. Hold the breath in until you come slowly down. Do this, alternating the legs, three times each side.

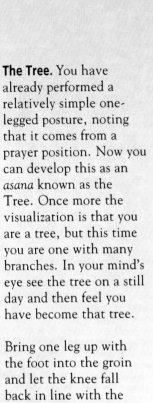

OVERCOMING FEAR OF FALLING

Do not be afraid of losing your balance if you are drawn into visualization. Providing you are relaxed, even if you stumble or fall you will not hurt yourself. Damage from falling is mainly as a result of tension. In any case this process will markedly reduce the chance of tumbling.

A LITTLE FURTHER STILL

The Back Body Stretch and the Cobra were chosen as two basic postures which could be seen to develop over the months. This does not, of course, mean that other postures do not develop in the same way, but by observing the ways in which you stimulate progress with these two, you can apply the same principles to others.

Back Body Stretch. Most people, when they begin to practise this stretch, content themselves with holding their ankles and calves. Before long they find they can hold their toes. Now is the time to explore the capacity to link the hands around the feet.

Remember that everyone's body is built differently and do not force the movements. However, with the right approach, great progress can be made. Make sure that as you stretch the arms up on the in-breath, you elongate the back and open up the spine as fully as possible. Make sure you do not lose this stretch as you begin to breathe out and move forward. The movement should be as effortless as a drawbridge coming down. Tension in the mind can put an undue strain on the lower back muscles and this can be damaging.

The stretch forward and down should continue the feeling of well-being. The more you enjoy this, the better the muscles and joints will respond.

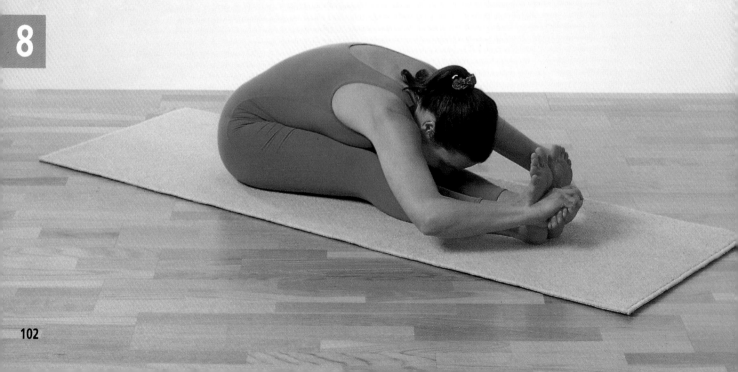

Always remember that in a very real sense the body wants to be used. Many medical practitioners confirm that one of humankind's major problems is called "disuse atrophy", or "If you don't use it, you lose it." There may be specific physiological reasons why you cannot perform certain postures fully, but don't fall back on the excuse that you are stiff.

· · · · · · · · · · · · · · · · · · · ·

CREATING ENERGY FLOW

In today's frenetic society, everyone lets themselves be dominated by time. The result is we achieve less, fail to do things properly and damage both mind and body.

If you lose yourself in postures such as these, the energy flows freely, the body benefits and you are stimulated mentally. You can get much more done in a day if you do each thing fully. These postures can be immensely helpful in this respect.

The Cobra. The same principles apply here. The back will follow the stretch to the front of the trunk and you will find the palms can move closer in, remembering at all times to keep the arms straight, with no bend at the elbows. If the legs and hips take the weight, the balance becomes comfortable and you can appreciate the sinuosity of the movement.

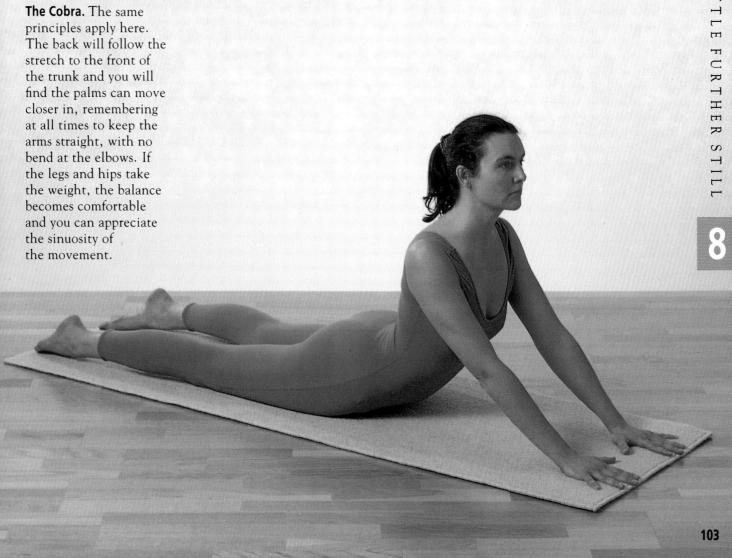

CONTINUING THE PROGRAMME

There are many people only too ready to tell you the "right way" to do something, although there is rarely a specific "right way". Some yoga teachers extol the virtue of performing each sequence every day. Others urge variety.

It is important to realize that what is offered in these pages is a series of examples: the final decision is yours. This decision should arise from tuning in more and more to the requirements of body and mind.

It takes some time to distinguish intuition from inclination. Avoid giving in to the "I don't feel like it today" syndrome, but realize that this feeling may direct you to a programme that meets the specific need of the moment.

POSTURES
The Tree offers an interesting posture development. The Simple Tree is a prayer – or meditative – position; the second a more specific balanced stretch. Do not, however, lose the meditative value in attempting the more advanced posture. Concentrate on balance, not imbalance, realize how much the mind directs the body.

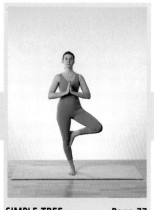

SIMPLE TREE   Page 77

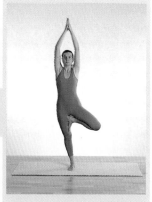

TREE   Page 101

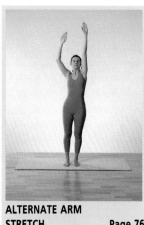

ALTERNATE ARM STRETCH   Page 76

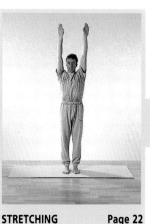

STRETCHING   Page 22

Spending some time on different aspects of stretching helps to clarify the advantages and to explain why apparently similar movements will produce a variety of results. If you clear your mind and accept the feedback, you will find significant differences.

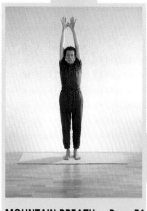

MOUNTAIN BREATH   Page 54

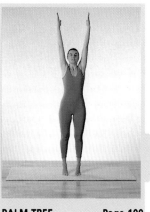

PALM TREE   Page 100

BREATHING
When clearing the air in the lungs with the "Ha" breath, add a further dimension by remaining down after the third exhalation. When no more air can be expelled; breathe gently through the nose and bend the arms, so that each hand holds the opposite elbow.

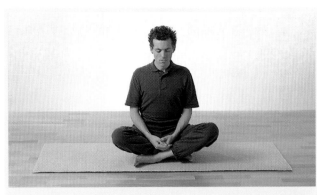

Page 37

Chronic pain can be diminished, even eradicated, by processes similar to the one with the clay. Develop the feeling that you do not need the discomfort and that you are taking it out of your body and placing it somewhere else, where it cannot return to you. The key to success lies in the degree of concentration.

VISUALIZATION

Remember that there are countless ways of visualizing. Provided you follow the basic rules, you can introduce your own concepts. Always be erect, always let the breath be quiet and rhythmical, and keep the eyes closed and the hands together on the lap.

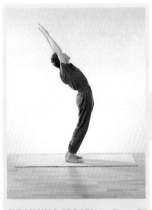

CLEANSING BREATH Page 55

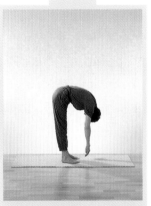

CLEANSING BREATH Page 55

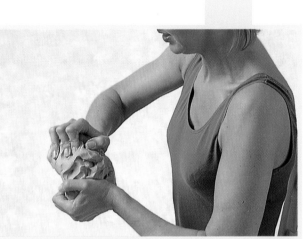

Page 97

Continue to breathe rhythmically and feel the head and shoulders come down a little as you breathe out. Let this be a natural stretch – do not tug. After two or three minutes, drop the arms again and, on an in-breath, straighten up, swinging the arms over the head and bringing them down by the side on the out-breath. This will enhance the suppleness of the lower back muscles.

MEDITATION

Pranayama techniques control the breath to control the mind. Once you have practised retaining the breath, this can be used as a preliminary to meditation. Breathing in, sitting on one's "cushion" of air and retaining the breath for a minute or so, will, once you are used to it, induce a feeling of calmness. Follow on immediately with a short period of meditation.

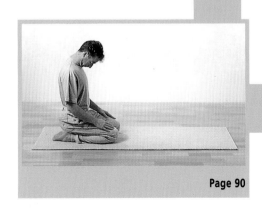

Page 90

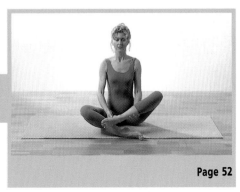

Page 52

CONTINUING THE PROGRAMME

8

DEVELOPING ASANAS

AIMS FOR THE MONTH

By now it will be obvious that you are developing quite slowly as far as the asanas are concerned. This is deliberate; it is better to learn to do a few things well, rather than a lot indifferently. Many people take up exercise programmes and other systems that offer all sorts of techniques, but very few keep them up for long, primarily because they are superficial. By its clear, slow integrated progress, yoga becomes a way of life and every aspect of living is enhanced as a result. This month you continue to bind all the strands of yoga together.

• •

STANDING BACK AND BODY STRETCH

Touching the toes is an exercise everyone performs as a child; some keep it up much later in life. However, most tend to "snatch" at it, thus jerking the neuro-muscular system, often doing more harm than good.

• • • • • • • • • • • • • • • • • • • •

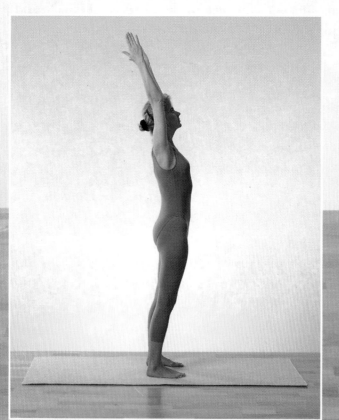

1 Stand with the feet some 12in (30cm) apart, arms by the sides. Breathe out, and, on the in-breath, swing the arms, quite slowly, into the air, lifting the trunk.

2 On the out-breath, swing forward, continuing to stretch and come down as far as you can, with the arms hanging.

If possible, let the fingers touch the floor, preferably, place the palms on the floor. Shake the head a little to make sure you are not holding tension in the neck. Breathing gently and slowly, hold the position for a minute or two, lengthening the time with practice.

Come up on an in-breath, reversing the whole process carefully and finish by bringing the arms to the sides as you breathe out.

3 To counter the forward stretch, link the fingers behind the back and, as you breathe in, swing back with the arms well away from the buttocks and with the knees a little bent.

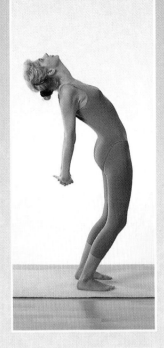

4 As you breathe out, come slowly back to the original position. Repeat steps 3 and 4 three times.

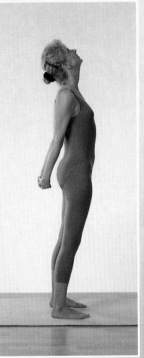

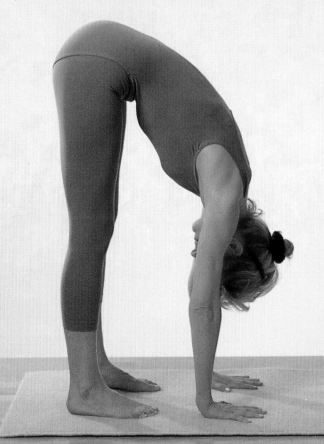

STANDING BACK AND BODY STRETCH

9

THE TRIANGLE

A *sideways bend was introduced earlier (see page 64). This was a relatively simple but effective movement that can certainly be retained in the programme. The best-known classical sideways bend posture is the Triangle, which you now move on to. The shoulders must remain parallel with the hips throughout. There is usually a tendency to twist the shoulders in order to achieve more, but this is wrong. The extent of the stretch can be improved gradually.*

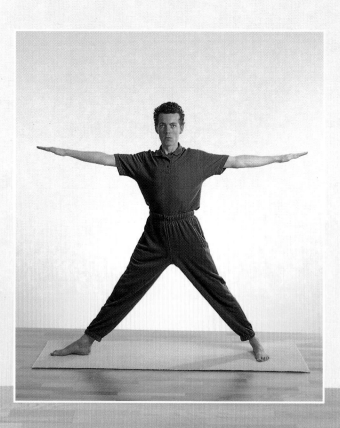

1 Stand with the feet quite wide apart (some 18in/45cm), the toes of the right foot pointing out at right angles, those of the left pointing slightly to the right. Breathing in, stretch the arms out to the sides.

2 As you breathe out, bring the right hand against your thigh and slide it down the calf while you lift the left hand into the air, turning the palm to face the front.

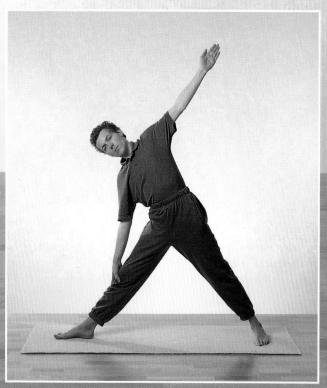

3 Look up at the hand in the air and let the right hand rest on, or hold, the ankle. Breathe quietly and hold the position. (In due course you may find you can place the right hand on the ground behind the foot.) When ready, come up on an in-breath, reversing the movement. Perform three times on each side.

IMPROVING

For an effective sideways bend, imagine you are an inverted pendulum. Before doing the posture it can be helpful to swing the trunk. Not only is this bend helpful to the spine, it balances the many functions within the trunk and also balances the muscle groups. Such spinal movements are particularly useful to people who play sports such as golf, tennis and cricket, that tend to exercise one side of the body only.

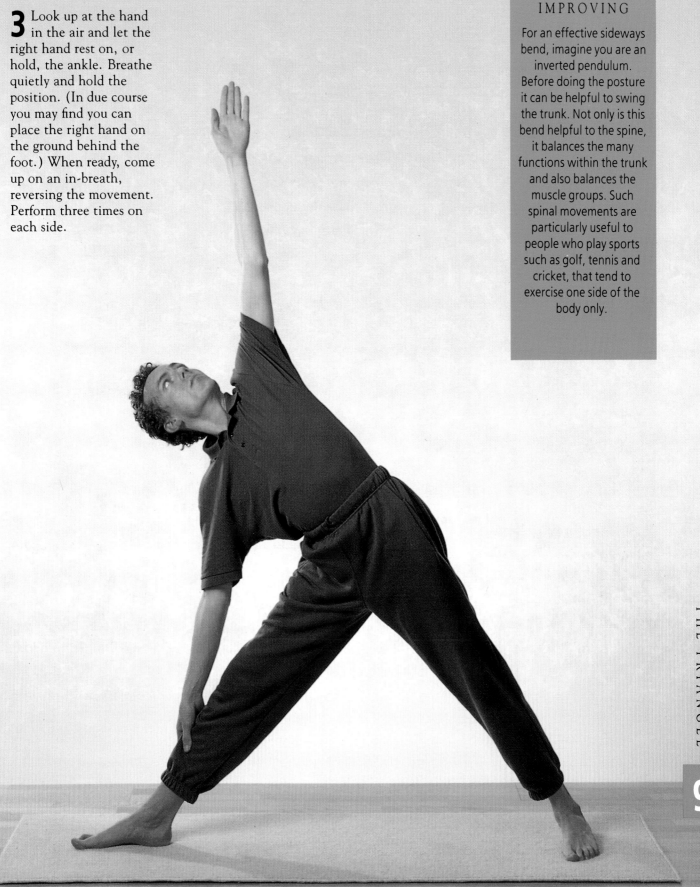

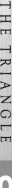

THE TRIANGLE

9

THE BOW

*The Bow is a strong posture and those who
are not naturally supple may find it difficult.
For such people – a considerable majority – it
is an interesting challenge in slowly but surely
letting things happen rather than striving after
them. To perform this posture effectively a
change in the normal approach to
breathing is important.*

1 Lie face down, with
the feet together,
head on the floor and the
arms by the sides, palms
up. Breathe out.

2 Breathing in, hold
the feet with the
hands and bend the legs
so the heels come in to
the buttocks.

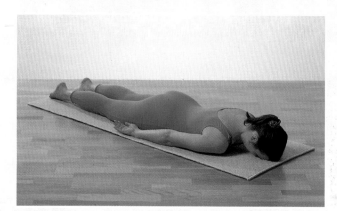

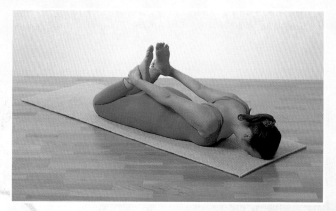

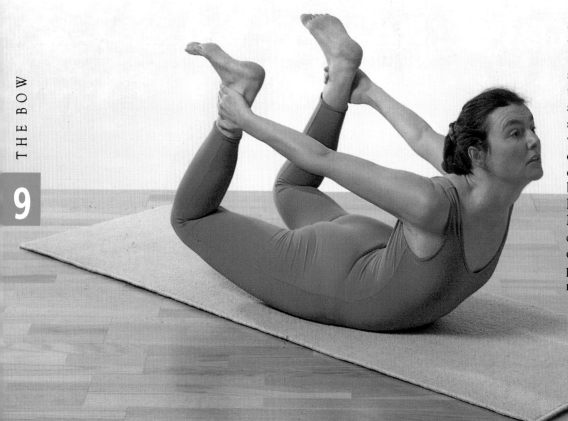

3 Breathe out, then
breathe in again and,
exactly at the moment
you breathe deeply out,
lift the head, shoulders
and chest, and pull on
the feet to lift the calves
and thighs off the floor,
so that you are resting on
your abdomen. Hold the
out-breath and then
come gently down again
before breathing in.
Repeat three times.
Making the movement
on the out-breath
ensures that the strong
pull is made on relaxing
muscles.

9

THE BOAT

This is a suitable counter posture to the Bow.
It requires an overall sense of balance.
Although many of the body's muscle groups
are put in tension, minimum effort is needed.

These postures present a special challenge, because while some strength and muscle tone is involved, the main constituent of success is a calm approach and an overall sense of balance. For many, these last two requirements provide the real challenge. It is worth reminding yourself that working towards these qualities will not only ensure good performance of the *asanas*, but will benefit you in many ways.

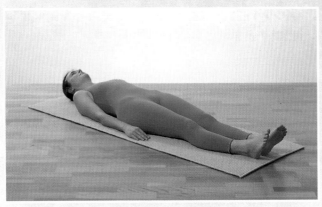

1 Lie on the back, feet together and arms by the sides, palms down.

2 Breathe out and, on the in-breath, swing the legs, straight into the air.

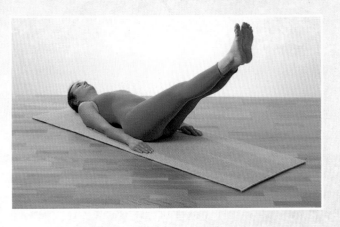

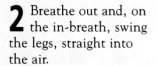

3 Stretch the arms in front of you. Finally, swing the trunk up, so that you are resting on the base of the spine, the arms outside the legs. Come down by reversing the movements on an out-breath. Repeat three times.

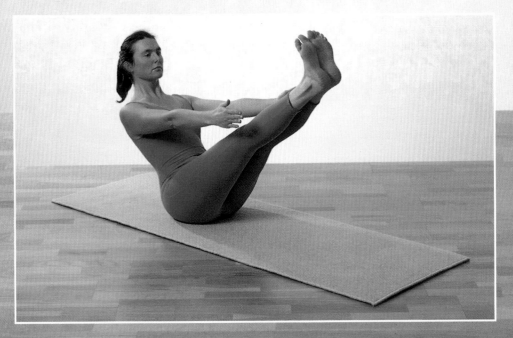

THE BOAT

9

111

Although the relaxation position has been shown and practised, it has not so far been analysed in detail. This is because you first have to become accustomed to relaxing in this way and then you can begin to remove pockets of tension. Relaxing is deceptively difficult because it involves letting go and "trying to relax" is a contradiction in terms. On these pages you can see the main areas where tension is apt to be retained. After consciously working on these for a while the body adjusts itself automatically and only rarely will it be necessary to go through the trouble spots.

Feet. When lying in relaxation the feet should be well apart, some 12-15in (30-40cm). This helps the leg muscles to relax. The ankles, too, need to relax, so the feet flop outwards.

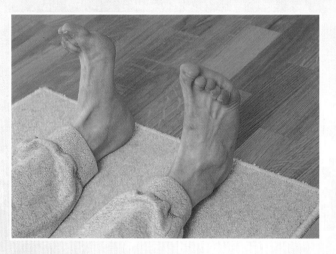

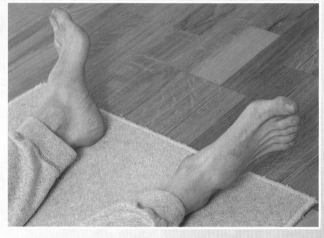

Back. Many people will find that when they are lying there is a gap between the lower back and the floor. This can be minimized by bending the knees, so the heels come into the buttocks, and by gently sliding the legs down again, at the same time consciously pressing the lower back against the floor.

9

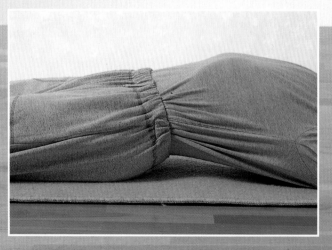

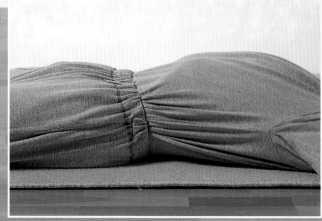

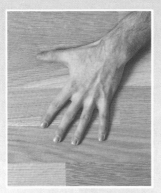
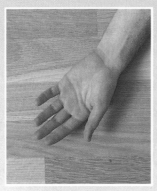

Hands. The arms should lie well away from the trunk and the hands rest comfortably, palms upward, not downward. It can be helpful to wave the hands and wrists loosely and then let them flop on the floor.

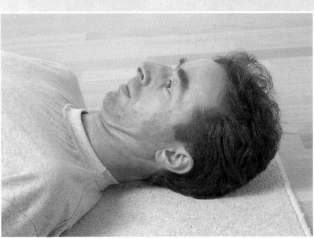

Head. The head should be in a straight line with the body, with the chin neither pressed in nor pulling away. A shake of the head will free the neck muscles and the shoulders should be consciously pressed against the floor and then relaxed.

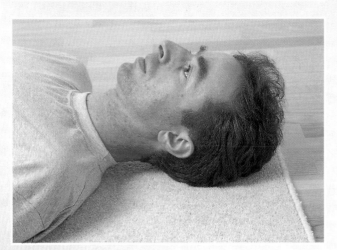

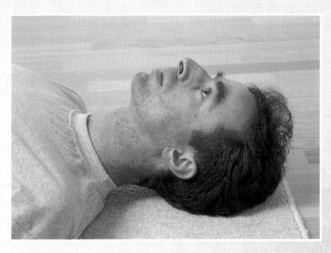

9

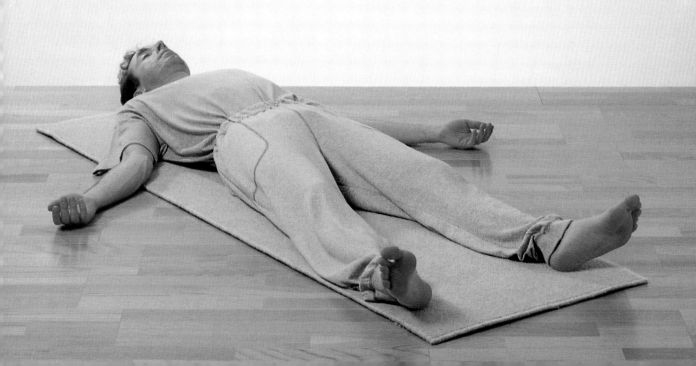

MORE STRENGTHENERS

Many people fail to realize that yoga asanas strengthen the body in a natural and effective way. This is a very different approach from body-building or similar techniques and it works equally well for both men and women. It is no part of yoga to create bulging or rippling muscles, but the essential strength of all parts of the body is improved considerably as part of a balanced programme.

The Mountain Breath.
This exercise which you have already been practising, combines deep use of the lungs and diaphragm with an upward stretch of the muscles of the trunk and arms. This variation involves a more lateral movement.

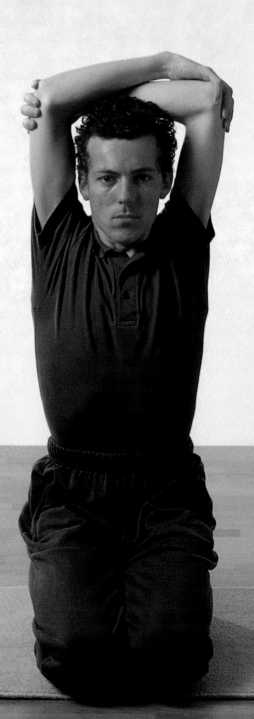

Sitting or standing, let the arms fall by the sides, palms and fingers open. Breathe deeply out and, on the in-breath, begin to stretch the arms out and up. As the arms come above the shoulder blades, begin to bend them until each hand is firmly gripping the opposite elbow. Make sure the arms are well back, in line with the back of the ears. Hold the position, keeping the breath in. When the impulse to breathe out becomes strong, begin to do so slowly, reversing the movement, until the arms are again by the sides. Repeat five or six times.

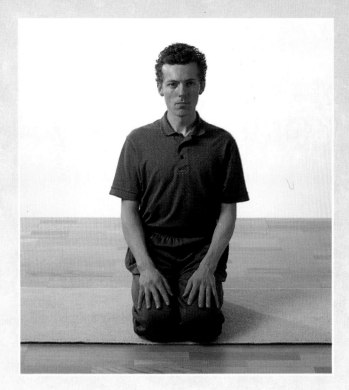

1 The Lion. This may look ferocious, but its aim is to provide an extremely strong therapeutic pressure, balanced by the subsequent relaxation. Sit erect with the hands on the knees or thighs and take a deep in-breath.

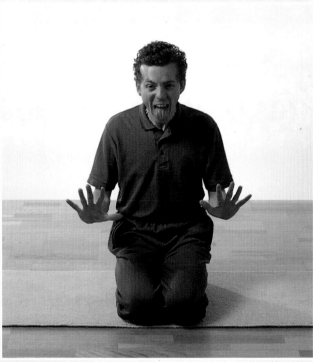

2 Breathe strongly out through the wide open mouth, expelling the air with a loud "Ha" sound. At the same time protrude the tongue until the tip touches the chin, and glare intensely at the tip of the nose, while tensing the fingers, hands and arms. Gradually let the muscles relax. Repeat three times.

The Tongue Lock. This exercise also provides strong balanced pressure. Sitting erect, breathe in through the nose. Holding the breath, force the mouth open wide, with the tongue placed limpet-like on the upper palate, until it comes away with a clicking sound. Repeat a number of times.

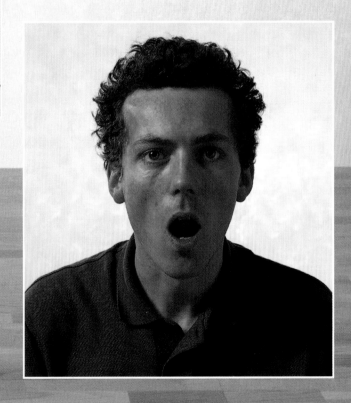

THE PEACE OF UNITY

The activities of the human brain are so
remarkable that you can hardly begin to
appreciate them. Many thousands of signals
are processed every second. Even when you
are in the state of dreamless sleep, the brain
continues to record and take in the
appropriate automatic action. But the brain is
the servant, not the master.

Once you take a step towards the mastery of
your own mind, you also take a step towards
a feeling of internal peace. When you begin to
calm the mind through meditation, you find
that the brain is constantly feeding you stray
and irrelevant thoughts and sensations. Often
the best way of handling these is to push them
away, gently and purposefully, so that you
can return to a state of concentration.

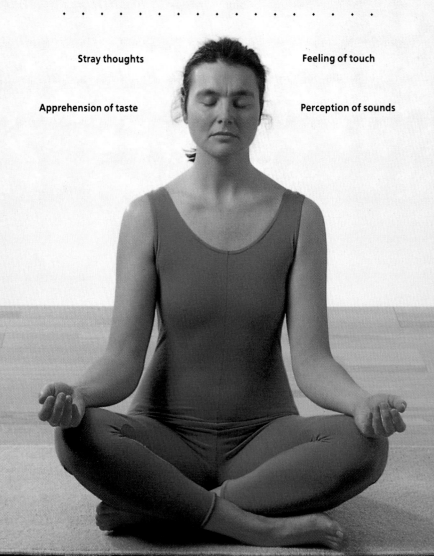

Stray thoughts

Feeling of touch

Apprehension of taste

Perception of sounds

PEACEFUL ACCEPTANCE

While pushing away ideas that are not required is often desirable, it can be just as successful to practise accepting them.

Try sitting quietly in the meditative pose, breathing slowly and gently, letting the feeling of calmness sweep over you. Then, when the brain begins to turn, accept the messages, even welcome them. Pay attention to each stray thought. Note carefully every sound. Become aware of any sensation of taste. Appreciate the feeling of touch: the clothes against the skin, the body against the floor.

The result will be similar to what happens when a naughty child tries to goad his or her parents into reaction. The more the child succeeds, the worse the problem becomes; the more the parents note, but do not react to, the child's naughtiness, the more the child feels a sense of anticlimax. Teasing is no fun any more and before long he or she gives up.

Letting the brain/mind know that you will accept or ignore its messages as you wish plays a significant part in helping to quieten it, and also in stimulating a deep internal feeling of well-being.

LEARNING TO SWITCH OFF

The various approaches to mental control should not be kept simply for specific sessions. Many a problem can be resolved by switching off for a short period – even a minute or two – before tackling it again. In the right surroundings and the right weather, we can all feel peaceful, but when you feel a sense of peace during periods of noise or confusion you know that you are making progress.

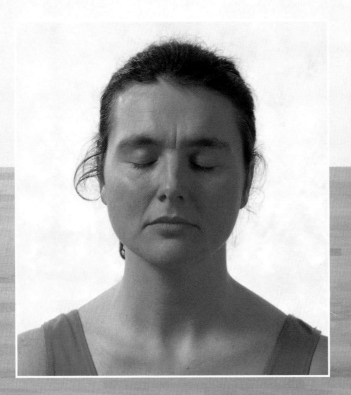

Whenever you sit quietly, in meditation, visualization or even in relaxation, take note of your face. Body language involves the way in which the facial muscles are used: not only do people screw their faces up against bright light, the wind or some other phenomenon, but they tend to do so in relation to problems. Become aware of your brow and allow any furrows to drop out. Relax the muscles around the eyes. Let the mouth and jaw be slack and ensure the tongue, too, is not tensed up against the palate. This simple process will be a positive aid to calmness, and it will also make you look younger and more attractive.

CONTINUING THE PROGRAMME

This month we focus on some stronger postures. Remember that such postures in yoga are not "show off" activities. If you find some of them beyond you, despite being in the right mental state and having advanced carefully and slowly, do not worry. Work away gently, but do not allow yourself to feel irritated, frustrated or upset: these emotions are damaging and will obstruct your goal.

Try to be dispassionate, and simply accept that this is your degree of performance for today. Remember, too, that human bodies vary considerably physically and that what is easy for one person is extremely difficult for another. Accepting genuine limitations is as important as overcoming mental inhibitions.

9

POSTURES

You have now advanced from a simple Side Bend to the classical Triangle. Both are still valuable. Never discard simple things: they all have their value. Do not fall into the trap of wanting to be "advanced". True humility is important.

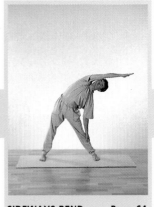

SIDEWAYS BEND   Page 64

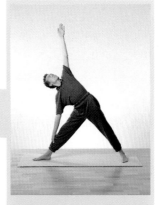

TRIANGLE   Page 109

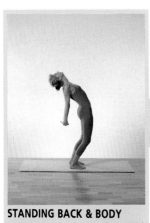

STANDING BACK & BODY STRETCH   Page 106

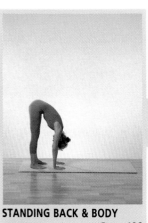

STANDING BACK & BODY STRETCH   Page 106

Having concentrated earlier on the sitting Back Body Stretch we now introduce the standing version. The combination of a genuine stretch with a relaxed state of mind remains vital. Muscles will bear a remarkable load if they are encouraged rather than tugged at.

It is important to keep practising the earlier Back Body Stretch and the Cobra. You will notice the improvement in your ability to perform these poses as the months pass.

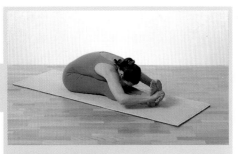

BACK BODY STRETCH   Page 102

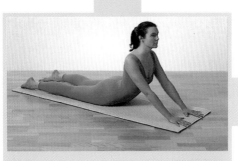

COBRA   Page 103

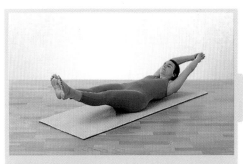

REVERSE CANOE   Page 35

The Bow and the Boat take you further into neuro-muscular control. As with so many of the *asanas*, the name of the posture can help in its performance. If you see these positions as challenging, or threatening, we shall create a wholly wrong approach, mentally and physically. If you visualize a bow or a boat, seek to become one with the visualization.

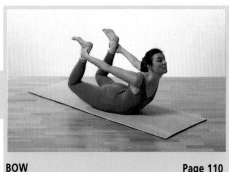

BOW   Page 110

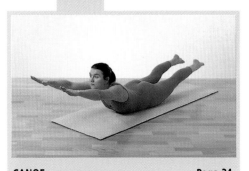

CANOE   Page 34

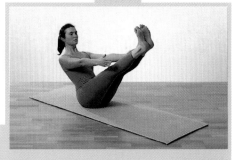

BOAT   Page 111

You have now developed a sequence of postures that will, among other things, develop control of the abdominal muscles.

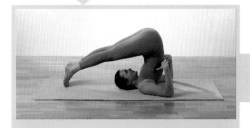

PLOUGH   Page 57

Both versions of the Plough remain valuable. Including inverted poses in a session provides balance.

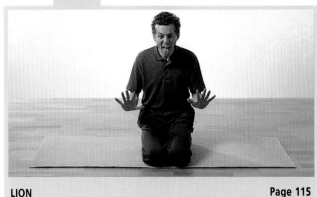

LION   Page 115

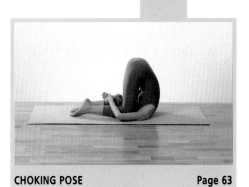

CHOKING POSE   Page 63

As your daily programme becomes more demanding, the integral holistic approach allows it to become more and more strengthening. A genuinely strong body arises from a genuinely calm mental state. Consider how many sportspeople experience physical problems, sometimes severe enough to end their careers.

MEDITATION
It may seem strange to have taken so long to introduce the idea that letting thoughts flit across the mind can help you to clear it, but you need to have experienced the annoying habit they have of intervening before you can be relaxed enough to deal with them in this way.

PROPORTION

AIMS FOR THE MONTH

The more involved you become with a subject, the more you take it seriously. In many ways this is excellent, but you need to keep a sense of proportion and to ensure that fun and lightness never lose their role. This is, after all, only another example of the need for balance. You are now nearing the end of your opening year, and it is time to leaven the progress with effective lightheartedness. The leading exponents of yoga in India – the swamis – all have a great sense of humour. This month, therefore, progress – both mental and physical – is maintained through knowledge, practice and enjoyment.

THE HULA HULA ASANA

This makes no pretence of being a yoga posture, but possibly the only reason it isn't is climatic. People living in hot climates tend to be more supple than those in the colder zones; their bodies are not always seizing-up against chill winds and pouring rain. Westerners need to counter the weather's effect.

1 Stand with the feet apart and place the hands on the hips.

2 Begin to gyrate the hips, as though doing a sexy dance or keeping a hula hoop in the air.

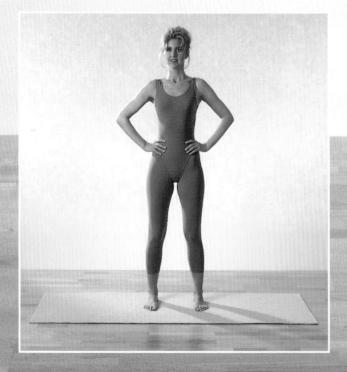

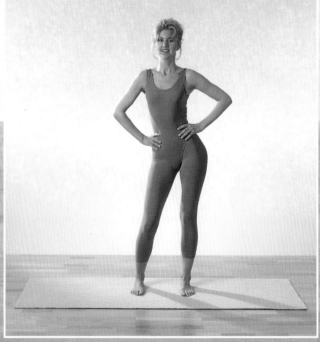

3 Sense the rhythm, speed up, slow down and at all times make the wiggle as wild as you can – have fun doing it. You will find your breathing adjusts itself to the movement.

If done with a sense of fun, this exercise will liberate the lower back, not only making it easier to perform the classical *asanas* for the spine, but also improving general suppleness. If it is performed too earnestly, the tension could pull a muscle; so let go and enjoy yourself. It's great to be a child again.

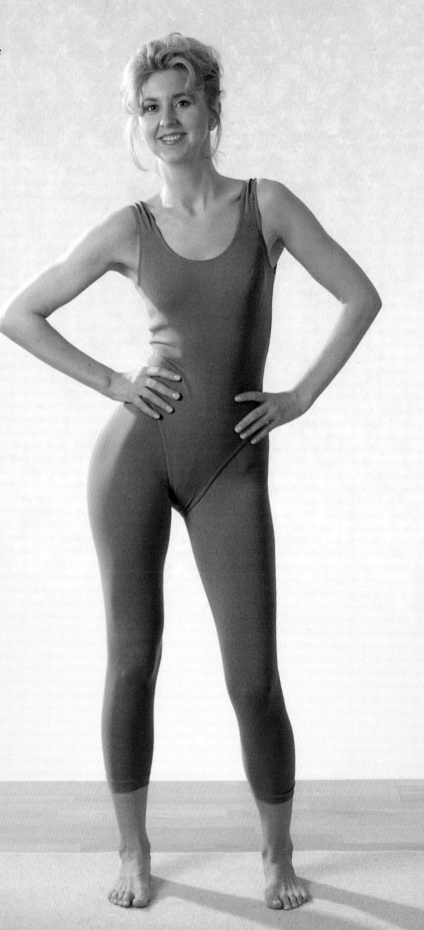

THE HULA HULA ASANA

10

THE HANUMAN POSES

Hanuman, *king of the monkeys, plays*
a beneficent role in Indian mythology.
These strong poses combine the use of the
breath with effective control of the muscles.

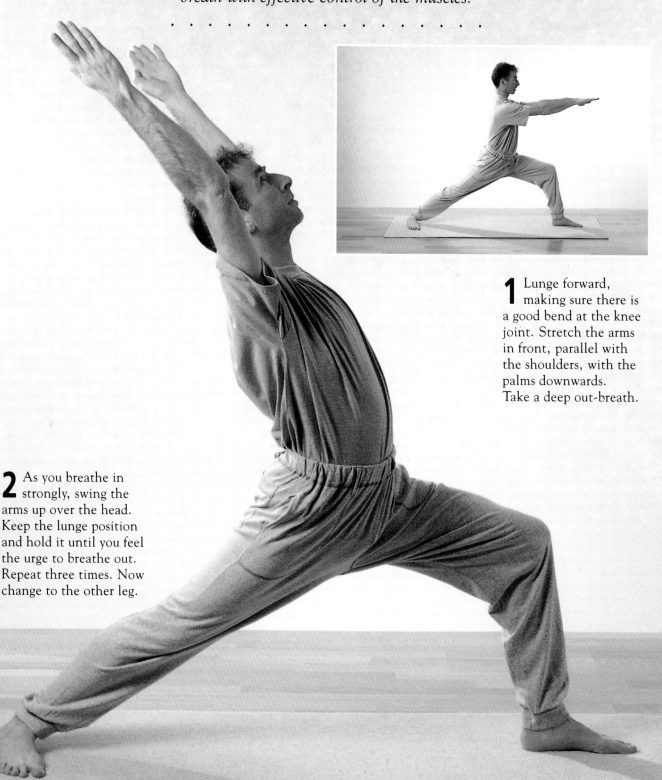

1 Lunge forward, making sure there is a good bend at the knee joint. Stretch the arms in front, parallel with the shoulders, with the palms downwards. Take a deep out-breath.

2 As you breathe in strongly, swing the arms up over the head. Keep the lunge position and hold it until you feel the urge to breathe out. Repeat three times. Now change to the other leg.

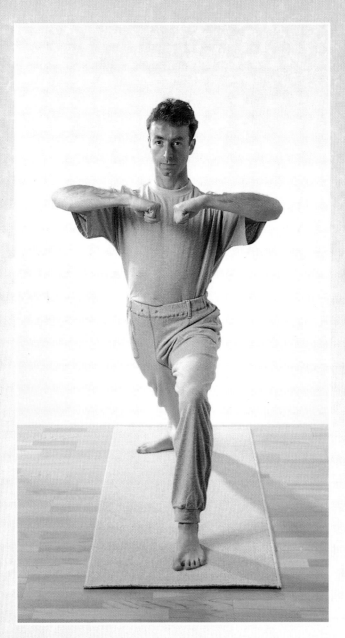

3 Lunge again, as in 1, but this time, as you breathe out, bring the clenched fists together (thumbs inside) with the knuckles almost touching.

There is a big difference between a forceful movement and a jerky one. Some of the injuries suffered by sportsmen are caused because they have not been trained to distinguish the difference. A strong movement in yoga is performed *naturally*: that is, without undue tension, and with the flow of the breath, and because everything about it has been accepted by the mind. Aim at slow, positive progress.

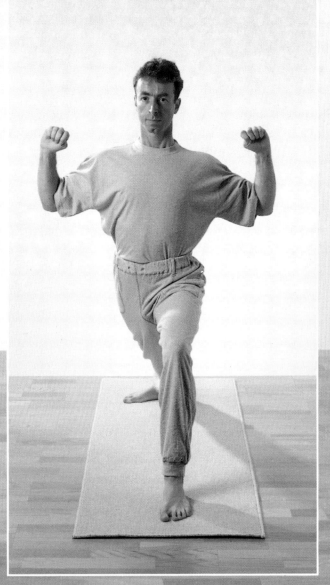

4 Once again breathing in strongly, swing the arms outwards so the chest is well expanded. Again hold the position; repeat three times and then change to the other leg. Repeat three times again.

THE HANUMAN POSES

10

The essential element of sitting correctly is the erect back. One of the images that most people associate with yoga is the Lotus Position, in which each foot rests on the opposite thigh. Children find this simple to do, but adults find it more difficult. When practising sitting postures, it is important to remember the knee is a hinge joint – it is not designed to rotate. Therefore it must be used carefully. The Lotus is best taught on a one-to-one basis and many people can advance well in yoga while still only sitting in a relatively simple cross-legged position. With gentle but persistent practice this can become balanced and comfortable.

1 To improve the cross-legged position, sit on the floor and take one ankle in both hands, while the other leg is bent in to the groin. Now use the hands to lift the ankle, while the leg muscles seek to pull down the knee. Practise for a few minutes with each leg. The movement needs to be rhythmical, not jerky.

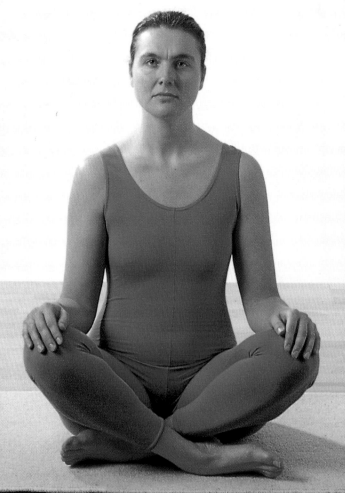

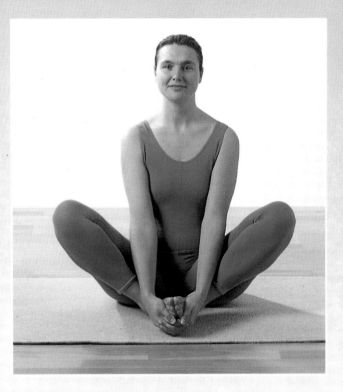

2 Now bring the soles of the feet together and bring the hands around the feet.

There are many views on the correct way to sit on the floor in yoga. If you intend to do so for some time it is sensible to place a folded-up blanket or a cushion under the buttocks.

While discomfort is often felt in the early stages, if you proceed correctly you will be rewarded with a growing feeling of comfort. Eventually you wonder how you came to sit any other way.

3 Holding the feet, move the knees up and down. This is often called a "butterfly" movement. You will feel the strain in the groin area, but if you maintain the rhythm and the feeling for the butterfly-like movement, the muscles will slowly accept the pressure and stretch sufficiently. When you have done this for two or three minutes, keep the soles of the feet together but place one hand on each knee and gently but firmly push it downwards. It will not be long before you notice a distinct improvement.

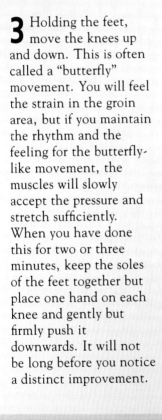

SITTING COMFORTABLY

10

125

BUILDING UP ENERGY

Energy, the be-all and end-all of existence, was discussed on page 83, where we pointed out how much misunderstanding there is about the matter. Oxygen plays a central role in human life, but it is not essential to all life. According to the philosophy of yoga, there has to be some basic force that is universal and upon which countless permutations are built. The ancient yogis called this force prana; the Chinese called it chi; Bergsen called it elan vital. Generally, it is translated as Life Force. You have already been practising working with this force: now, with the aid of a friend, you can experience it more precisely.

1 The natural breathing process is for the bottom ribs to move up and out on the in-breath, stretching the diaphragm, and to fall back on the out-breath, the abdomen and chest remaining still. Some people claim that, to use the lungs effectively, the abdomen should also expand and contract with the breath.

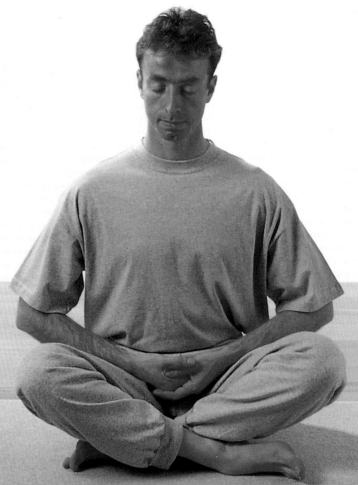

The two forms of breathing shown allow the lungs to be used equally well, so the changes in strength cannot be caused by oxygen. The difference comes from stimulating the electrical flow down the nervous system, a factor discovered many years ago. Breathing naturally, therefore, you generate your own electrical force, upon which all other aspects of energy depend.

BREATHING CORRECTLY

Most youngsters have natural poise and breathe as nature intended. Our way of life, with its tensions and pressures, knocks this out of us quite early. Once you have restored the natural posture, you can improve the breathing. To start with you need to practise, even if only briefly, quite frequently. This will be recorded on a "floppy disc" in the brain – in other words you establish a reflex action that will come into force as required.

2 Get a friend to help you and, before you begin, put one arm out to the side, tense the muscles and ask your friend to push it down firmly. Take half a dozen deepish breaths, allowing the abdomen to expand as you breathe in. Now get your friend to check the tone of the arm muscle once more. It will have gone quite weak.

Next, take a similar number of deepish breaths with the abdomen and chest still and the bottom ribs moving out and back (as you have been practising already). Get your friend to try once more: your arm will have strengthened markedly.

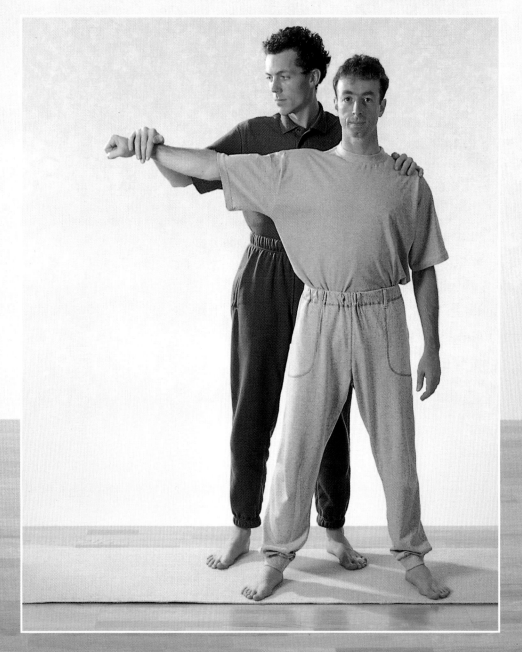

10

CONTINUING THE PROGRAMME

It is not possible to impose feelings of vitality, peace, joy – they all come from within. The "Continuing the Programme" spreads are an aide memoire rather than detailed working sheets. If attention this month is centred on sitting it does not, of course, mean that steady practice of all the other aspects should be abandoned.

People who know little else about yoga have often heard of the Lotus position, which involves placing each foot on the opposite thigh. When we were young children, most of us could do this easily, showing that it is in no way unnatural. However, as we grow up, the nature of the lives most of us lead makes us in some ways stiffer and stiffer.

As a result, the Lotus is not offered in this book. Those who can achieve it without damaging the knee joints are free to do so, but it is only one of a number of effective sitting positions.

Bad posture distorts the body, putting wrong strains and pressures on joints, ligaments, muscles and so on. This physical distortion is reflected in the brain, which passes on the messages of discomfort to the mind. This discomfort is not merely registered physically, it also begins to damage our outlook generally.

POSTURE
Sitting, standing and walking upright are natural activities for humankind, central to body design or development. As a result, an upright posture is the most comfortable way, for everything is in balance.

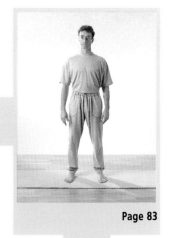

Page 83

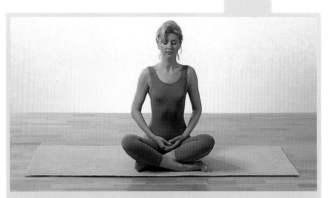

Page 72

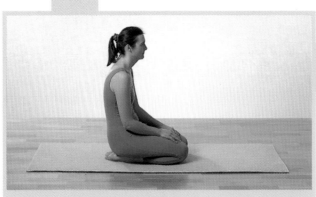

Page 42

Taking time to restore good posture is important in every way. Attention to standing posture is important, but it will tend to follow the posture we adopt when sitting. Getting that right is therefore of primary importance.

10

Sitting on the heels is quite simple. If the muscles in the ankles have tensed up, they will stretch back quite easily if they are trained in short, steady bouts. The feeling of discomfort will disappear quite soon in the majority of cases.

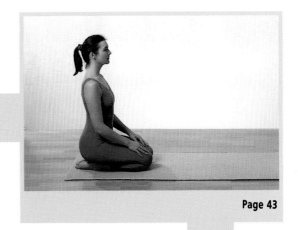

Page 43

Sitting cross-legged on a cushion or folded blanket is generally advisable. The muscles in the groin will also relax considerably if they are allowed to do so. Remember, they can be encouraged to do so with gentle hand pressure.

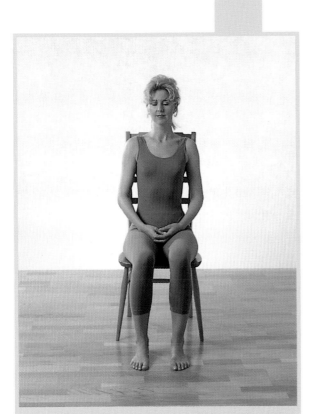

Page 38

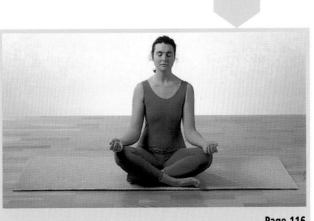

Page 116

SITTING
You can sit effectively in any reasonably well-designed chair. If the back of the chair does not provide good support, sit up and do not lean against it.

Once you have acquired the art of sitting and standing naturally, any other position seems irritating and uncomfortable.

10

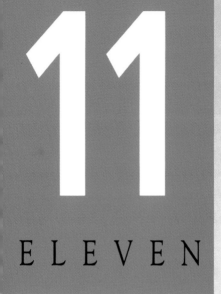

CENTRING – BECOMING ONE
AIMS FOR THE MONTH

An often used expression when mind and body are not functioning together is "out of sync". In this state it is easy to break things or misjudge distances; you cannot "think straight" and breathing becomes disturbed. There are, of course, prosaic explanations of what is happening, but normally no-one knows why. At this point in your practice a simple understanding of human synchronization is important.

THE BODY'S SHEATHS

The yogi sees the body as made up of a series of sheaths, superimposed one on the other. When life is balanced and harmonious these fit together closely and life functions as a co-ordinated whole. However, all too often the layers do not fit together and life becomes "disconnected". There are five of these sheaths; the first is the physical body, nourished by the food we eat; the second is the air we breathe, without which there is no life; the third, the storage and co-ordination functions of the brain; the fourth, the mental process, which gives us the opportunity to discriminate and exercise free will, even if this is only to a limited degree; the fifth is the link with universal consciousness, which results in many people having an occasional glimpse of one-ness, an ecstatic moment.

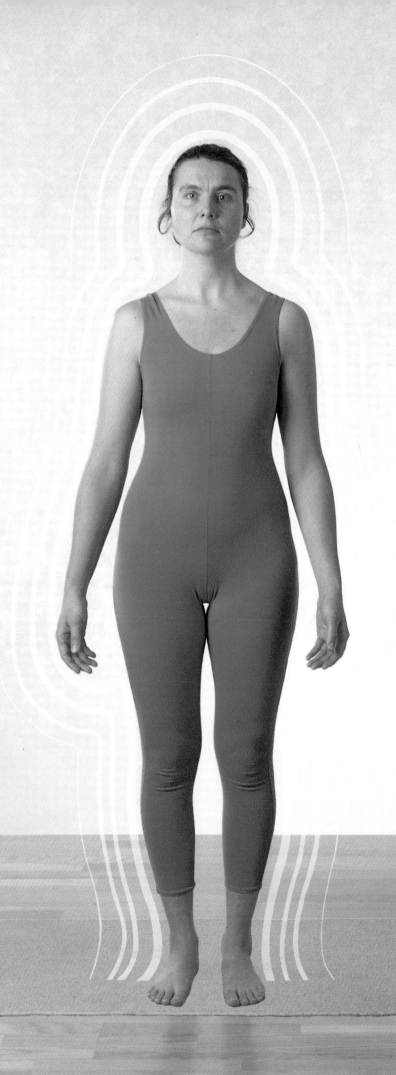

It is helpful to build up the realization of the various layers of consciousness that make up a human being. All aspects of yoga are directed towards the creation of an harmonious whole.

The sheaths can form an ideal subject for contemplation when you are sitting quietly, but there is no reason why you should not bring them to mind at other times. Just being aware of them is a step towards balance.

Thinking about the complexity of existence is helpful. While you can hardly begin to understand it, the realization that you are immersed in a sea of waves, vibrations and resonances helps in the vital process of knowing that you are a part of an immense whole, rather than an isolated unit.

THE TRIPOD

This inverted posture looks difficult, but it isn't, provided that instructions are followed carefully and the various aspects of your being are allowed to function together. It is, in fact an ideal posture to ensure that the five human sheaths are functioning together.

1 Come down on all fours, with the arms straight, palms down and facing forwards at shoulder level and at shoulder width.

2 Place the crown of the head on the floor so that it forms the apex of an equilateral triangle, with the hands as the bottom corners. Be quite sure you have the triangle right.

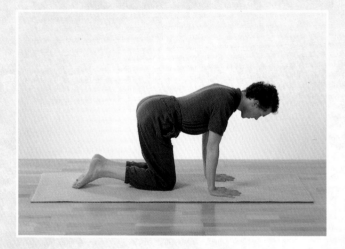

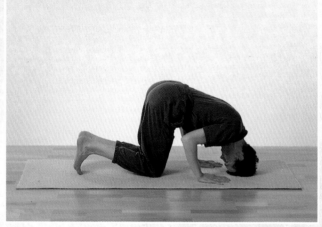

3 Bend the arms so that they are at right angles at all points. Place the right knee on the corresponding elbow.

4 Place the left knee on the corresponding elbow and balance comfortably breathing calmly and allowing the mind to maintain the quiet decision to hold the posture. Retain it for as long as you are comfortable.

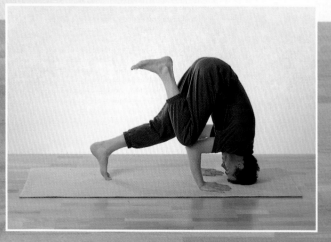

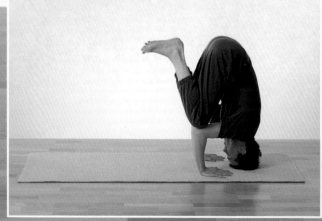

THE SCISSORS

One of the most valuable stretching asanas, the Scissors needs to be held for several minutes to be effective. Among its many benefits is a valuable extension of the sciatic nerve. As ever, the careful, calm mental process is basic.

In our pace-ridden society, there is a tendency to get things over and done with, but this desire to get on becomes exhausting and creates a feeling of dissatisfaction. One of the pleasures of developing yoga *asanas* is the satisfaction that grows steadily with working slowly and being able to hold static positions for an increasing length of time.

1 Lie on your back, feet together, with the arms stretched out to the sides, palms down. Breathe rhythmically and, as you breathe in, stretch the right leg up into the air.

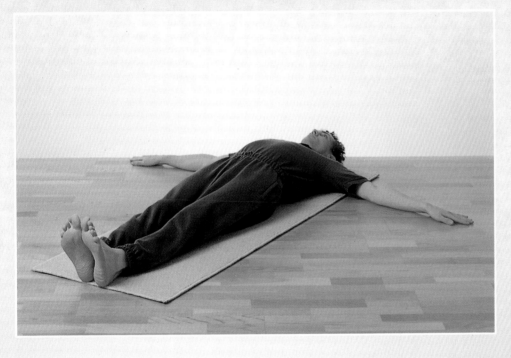

2 On the out-breath, bring the leg across the body, twisting the hips but keeping the shoulders firmly on the floor. Turn your head to the right as the leg comes down, straight, to the left. Relax as fully as you can and let it come down slowly, aided by the relaxation of a slow out-breath. If the leg does not touch the floor it does not matter.

Let the rhythm of your breath govern everything: the body will respond and the mind will quieten. Hold the pose for several minutes, then bring the right leg back and repeat with the left leg.

THE SCISSORS

11

CAT AND DOG

By now you are fully aware of the benefits of the Cat pose. Not only does it benefit the spine and the trunk, it is also a pleasing sensuous movement that makes you feel good. At this stage, you can add the Dog stretch, which benefits legs and ankles.

1 By now, when you do the Cat (see page 24) you are achieving much more spinal movement in the initial process. With the in-breath, drop the back, open the chest and swing up the head and neck.

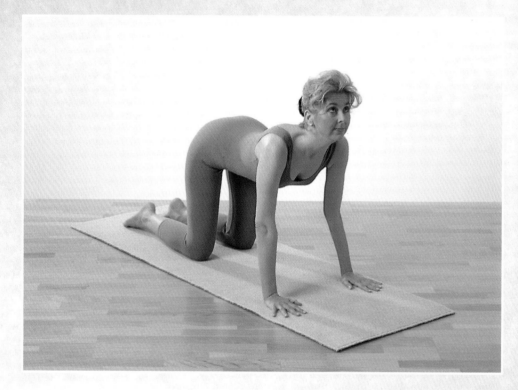

2 Breathing out, arch the back fully, with the head coming down firmly between the shoulders. Spine and trunk muscles are not only more mobile but the controlled movement strengthens them effectively.

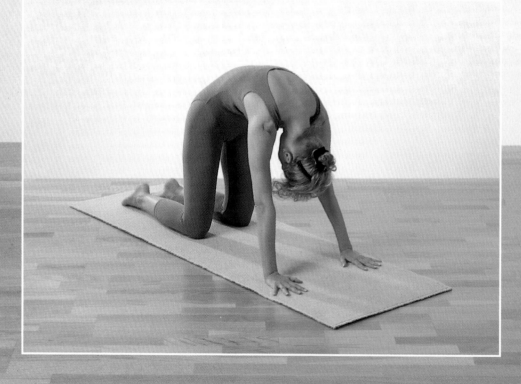

11

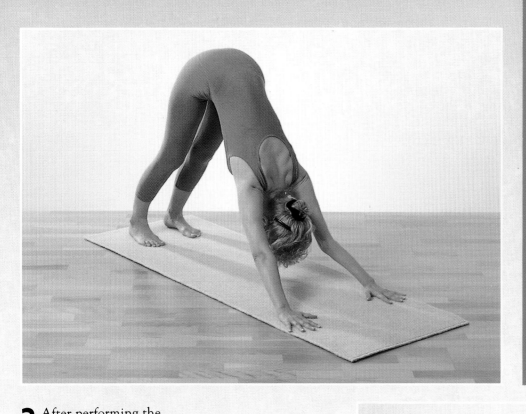

Two factors are responsible for a great deal of our back problems: failure to use the trunk effectively and making sudden, jerky movements. The slowly controlled sequence of yoga *asanas* not only enhances mobility of the spine, it also encourages the elasticity of the muscle groups, and promotes overall mobility, including mental agility. The stiffer you are physically, the less likely it is that your brain will work well.

3 After performing the initial movements several times, straighten the legs on an out-breath, thrusting the buttocks into the air.

4 Now bend alternate knees, raising the heel to do so, pressing the other foot firmly against the floor. Leg and ankle muscles are strengthened accordingly.

5 Finally, sink back on to the floor, forehead touching it, the arms lying by the sides, palms up, either side of the feet. Relax for a minute or two.

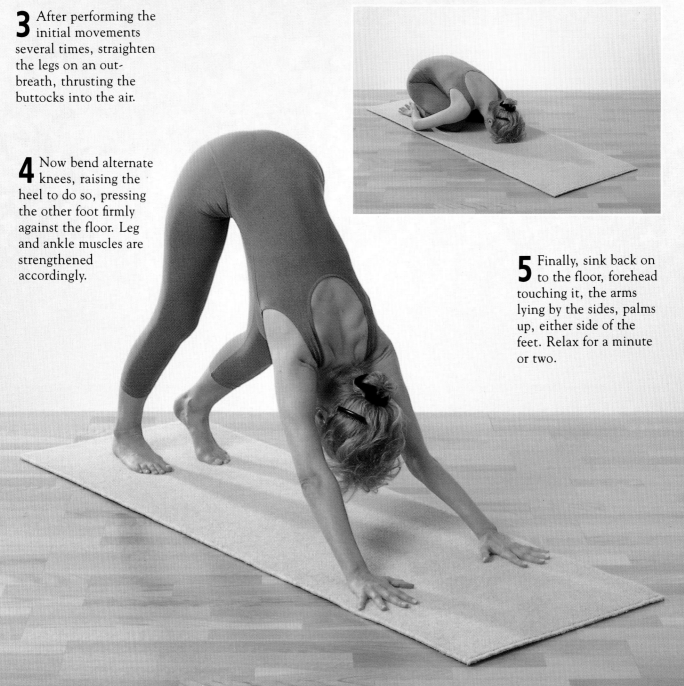

CAT AND DOG

11

DEVELOPING THE SHOULDER STAND

*Once a posture such as the Half-shoulder
Stand (see page 44) has been correctly
practised for some time (remember to take
much of the pressure on the shoulders and not
on the nape of the neck), you can move on to
variations that will add considerably to
the overall balance of life.*

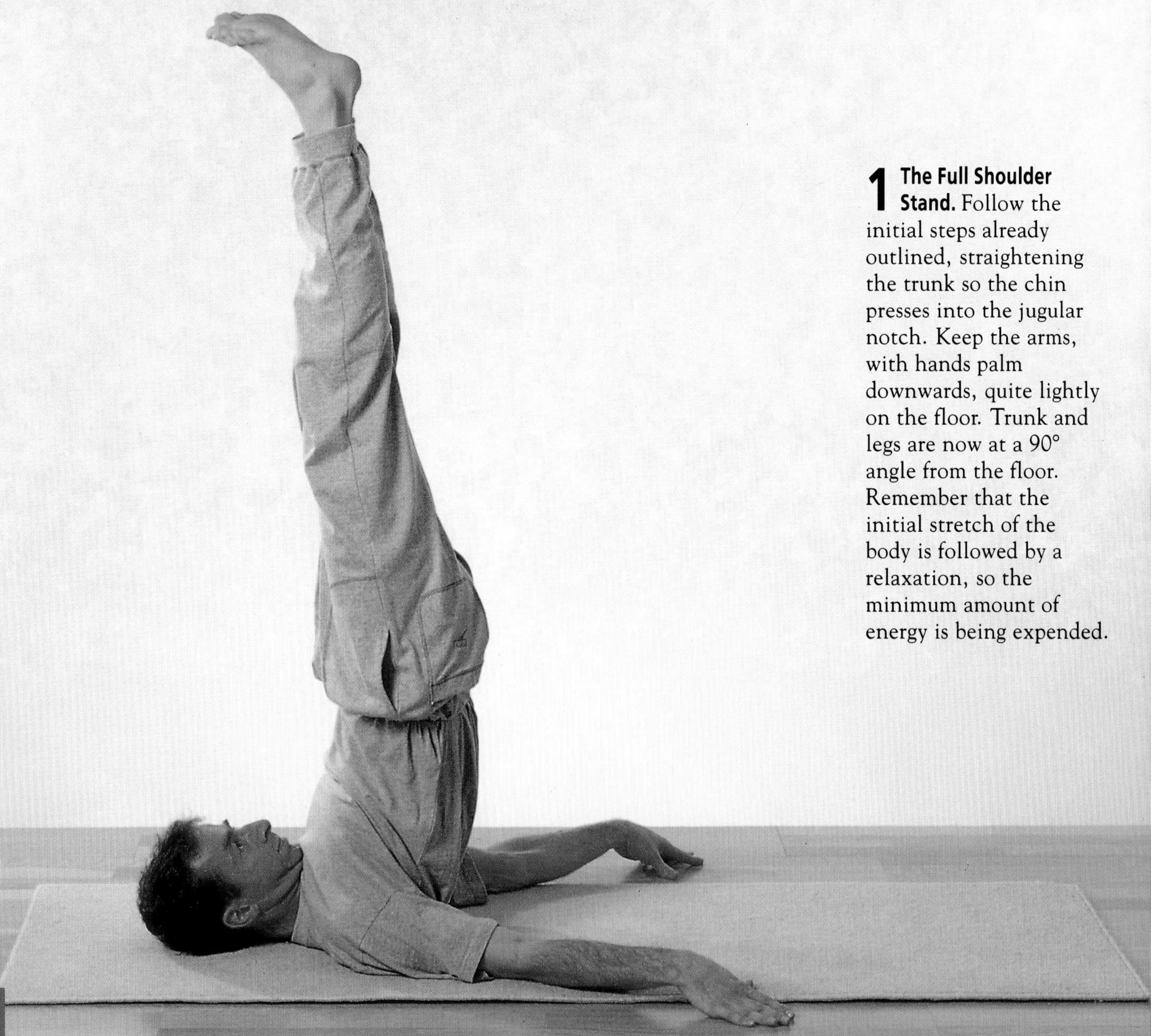

**1 The Full Shoulder
Stand.** Follow the
initial steps already
outlined, straightening
the trunk so the chin
presses into the jugular
notch. Keep the arms,
with hands palm
downwards, quite lightly
on the floor. Trunk and
legs are now at a 90°
angle from the floor.
Remember that the
initial stretch of the
body is followed by a
relaxation, so the
minimum amount of
energy is being expended.

11

2 Bring the hands lightly into the small of the back and then, as you breathe out, swing one leg down over your head – straight – aiming to bring the toes on to the floor. If you cannot immediately reach the floor, do not worry. Take your time and let the weight of the leg bring it down, with the muscles relaxed. Bring it back up on an in-breath and repeat with the other leg. Repeat as many times as you find comfortable.

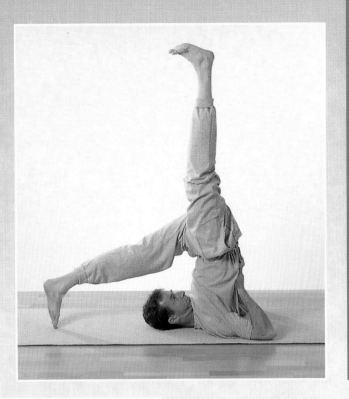

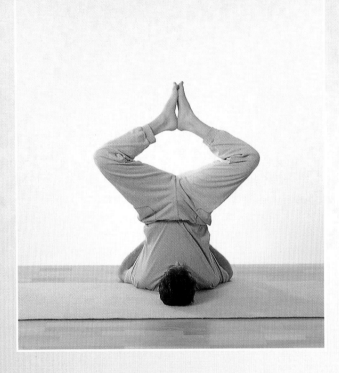

3 Still with the hands in the small of the back, bend the knees outwards and bring the soles of the feet together, also on an out-breath. Straighten on an in-breath. Repeat two or three times.

4 Finally, remove the arms from the back and straighten them by the sides, palms against the thighs. Let the legs move a little forward to maintain balance, but keep this movement as small as possible. Hold while you feel comfortable, breathing quietly and let a feeling of peace suffuse both mind and body. Before you come down, bring the arms back on the floor behind you to take the body's weight and let the legs swing slowly down to the floor. Relax for a minute or two.

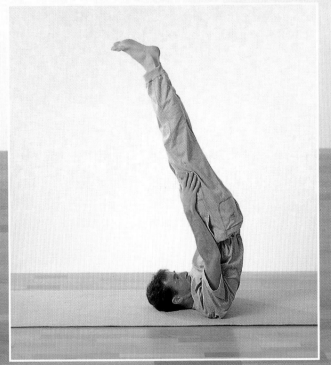

SPOT ENERGIZATION

Working constantly with the combination of body, energy, brain, mind and consciousness, increases the ability to control more fully many aspects of life. As you know, by visualization, it is possible to enhance the flow of body energy and, if this has been practised steadily, results will already be noticeable. Now you can move on to relieving and healing specific areas that give trouble.

First, bear in mind the fact that every problem has a mental link, as well as a physical one. If a part of the body is damaged in an accident, the brain sometimes links that damage with some mental difficulty such as fear, anger or worry, for example. This linking heightens tension, both mental and physical, which hampers the healing process, setting up blockages that prevent nutrients, anti-bodies and so forth getting through to the right area. A calm mental approach (remember

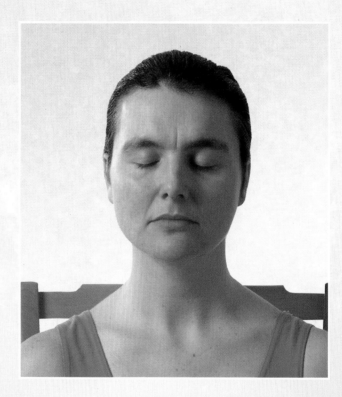

how the modelling clay imagery can release resentment and frustration) needs to be linked with an enhancement of body energy, to stimulate a flow of energy that will relax the body and allow the healing process to flow naturally.

The flow of breath – which is life itself – is at the core of this flow of energy. By now you know how to sit effectively, how to breathe slowly, calmly and rhythmically and how to let the mind dwell on the concept of energy and of healing.

For the sake of illustration, imagine you have injured a knee. Recovery from the injury is a natural body process, but even the very best medical attention does not in itself heal, it encourages the body's own ability to heal. This is a basic process, wholly without side-effects. It is also part of what could be called "body design", as it is central to the whole concept of consciousness.

Damage to a part of the body results in tension and a feedback of "discomfort messages" to the brain. This in turn, can result in negative messages being fed back from the brain to the damaged part, delaying or even preventing the process of healing. The mind, however, has immense power and if, with great concentration, we make sure that it sends strong opposing messages, the brain will accept these and act upon them.

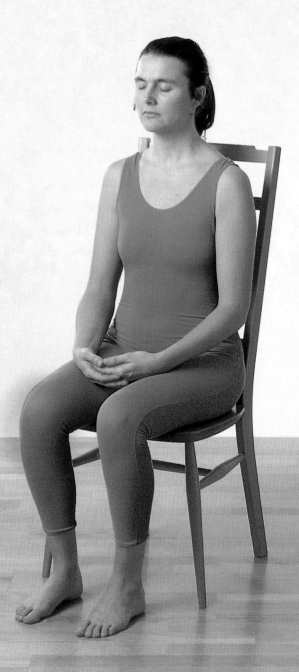

Sit in a chair, or on the floor, in the correct position, with the eyes closed. Pay attention to the quiet flow of your breath. Do not rush. After a short while, follow the process of feeling the energy in the breath flow to the top of the head as you breathe in and down through every part of the body as you breathe out. Feel the muscles in the face relax and then every part of the body responds to this slow, gentle flow. Before long the whole body will feel warm and tingling.

Focusing
Now take your mind to the part of the body that is causing trouble and from now on let each out-breath flow through it. Disregard the rest of the body. If it is a knee that is troublesome, let the mind dwell just on that knee and nothing else. Each time you breathe out, feel the warm energy flow through the knee: feel it radiating, tingling. Let no other thought intervene; you are wholly concerned with the flow of energy and the damaged knee. You will sense the tension diminishing as the circulation improves and the essential health flow is resumed.

Timing
Spend at least ten minutes a time on this, building up to 15 or 20. Do not expect a miracle, but be aware of steady progress. The speed of recovery will depend on a number of different factors, so be patient.

SPOT ENERGIZATION

11

CONTINUING THE PROGRAMME

Inverted postures have always played a central role in yoga. That this is natural can be seen from the fact that almost all energetic, healthy children love to do handstands!

There are many reasons for spending a little time upside down; a practical one is providing a useful counter to the constant process of gravity.

Inversion is stimulating, mentally and physically. However, proceed with common sense and, if you have blood pressure or heart problems, consult a well-qualified teacher first.

POSTURES

The Shoulder Stand is sometimes called the Topsy-Turvy pose. By taking your time and establishing a real feeling of mental and physical balance, you can move from a relatively simple position to holding the pose on the shoulders, without the support of the arms. Do remember to keep the shoulders free from tension and let them take the bulk of the weight.

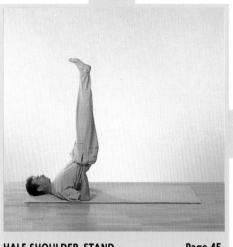

HALF-SHOULDER STAND   Page 45

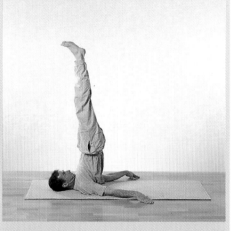

SHOULDER STAND   Page 136

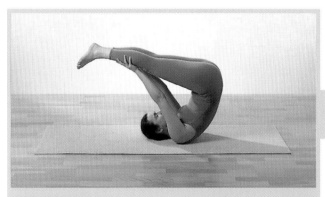

POSE OF TRANQUILITY   Page 56

The Pose of Tranquility and the Plough also provide a variety of benefits. Maintaining control at all times is most important. Never fall out of these or any other postures. The arms, placed on the ground, provide effective leverage.

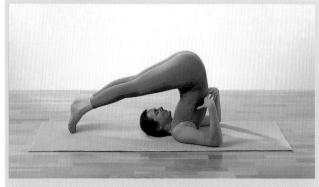

PLOUGH   Page 57

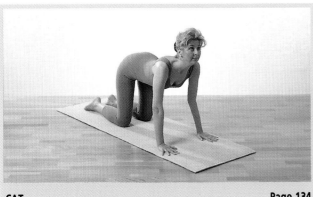

CAT Page 134

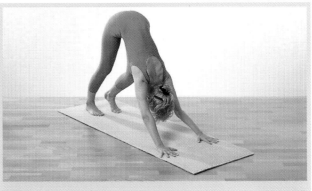

DOG Page 135

The Cat-to-Dog is not strictly an inverted posture, but its value is not dissimilar. Remember how easily and freely cats and dogs stretch. What they can do, you can do too.

The late Swami Sivananda, a doctor before he became a yogi, declared, "It takes 40 muscles to frown and only 15 to smile. Why waste your energy?"

As you become more aware through the practice of yoga, one aspect of this awareness is seeing how energy is wasted. Try to pull a cork out of a bottle and realize how you tense up the muscles of your face, although the latter plays no role in pulling out the cork. This wasted energy seems unimportant at the time, but it adds up. Over any single day you are likely to waste quite a substantial amount, and you wonder why you feel so tired. To achieve the maximum with the least tension, mentally and physically is central to the art of living.

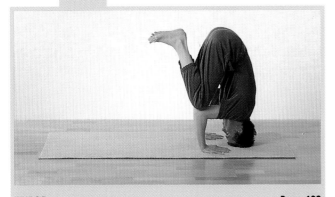

TRIPOD Page 132

The Tripod is an important lesson in precision. Forming the equilateral triangle and seeing that the arms make 90° angles are essential. This posture helps greatly in body awareness.

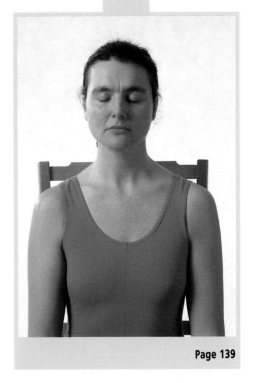

Page 139

11

FITTING POSTURE TO NEED

AIMS FOR THE MONTH

It will have become apparent that yoga is not simply a system in which you follow a standard pattern. It is the process of self-realization and therefore the principles have to be grasped and then adapted to each individual's needs. As you come to the end of your first year of practice, you should be aware that the development lies in your own approach. While yoga teachers can help, real knowledge lies within you. Through quiet harmony and the development of the capacity to be still, this knowledge becomes apparent.

CONTROLLING STRESS

We have already considered responses to the everyday ups-and-downs of life; now the time has come to consider this aspect somewhat more deeply. A common statement is, "One person's stress is another person's challenge." We cannot dodge the challenges of life, but we can control our response to them.

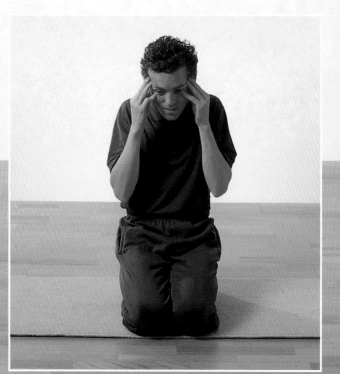

While, when life seems to be getting too much for us, we may outwardly seem to be coping, in fact many things are happening at the psychophysical level that can be extremely damaging. Respiration is affected, the body's neuro-muscular system is tensed and, in turn, organs are hampered from working properly.

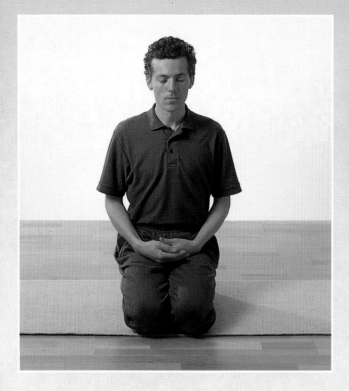

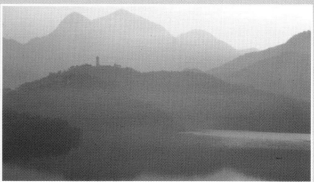

The brain responds according to the most effective impulse it receives. It is for this reason that meditative and visualization techniques have demonstrated human beings' remarkable capacity to achieve calmness even when things seem to be going badly wrong. You can push away the feeling that things are crushing you by sitting and visualizing a beautiful sunrise. You "see" the light appear in the sky, then the sun, slowly making its way into the heavens, with beautiful golden-red light all around. The more you develop this inward picture, the more the feeling of pressure will recede.

Practices such as meditation and visualization apart, *asanas* can be used to overcome mental problems, providing they are approached correctly. If you feel disturbed, for example, remember the Pose of Tranquility (see page 56). Its name describes its purpose and if you push disturbing thoughts away and give yourself to this inverted position, a great feeling of calmness will ensue.

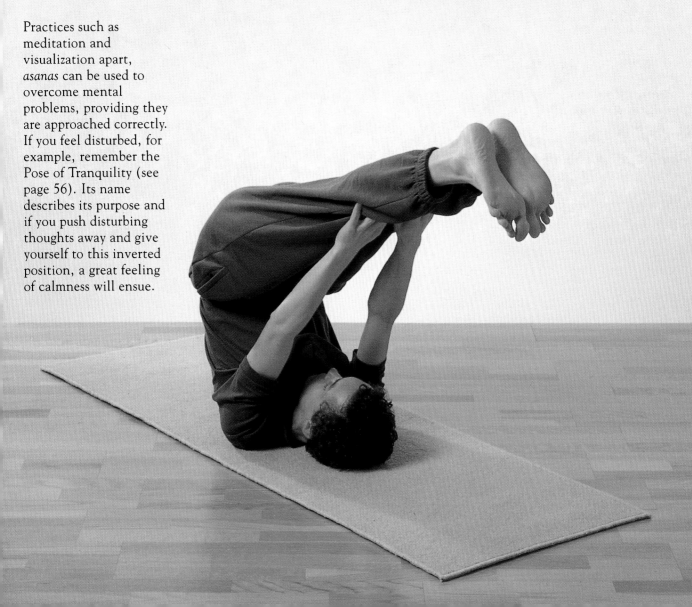

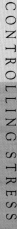

12

THE THERAPY OF LOVE

The central importance of love in life is undeniable. Because people tend to compartmentalize their lives, they often associate love with human relationships alone – even just with sexual activity. But there are no boundaries to love: love of life itself, love of beautiful things and love of God are all aspects of the same central feeling. The effect of love upon the body is very noticeable: a person who feels unloved is tense, sharp, brittle, while someone feeling the emotion of love is relaxed, soft and warm. Love is a much greater experience than that of immediate relationships, and you can use this wonderful feeling to enhance your health. This will, in turn, enhance the feeling!

1 You have already developed your performance of the Back Body Stretch, by working slowly but progressively. Now you move it wholly into the area of beneficial visualization. Perform the posture precisely as before. When you are as comfortably stretched as you can, become aware of the rhythm of your breath and, after a minute or two, see, in your mind's eye, someone you love, in front of you and stretching out their hands to reach yours. Choose any loving image: relation, friend, Jesus Christ, the Lord Krishna. Stretch forward to hold the proffered hands.

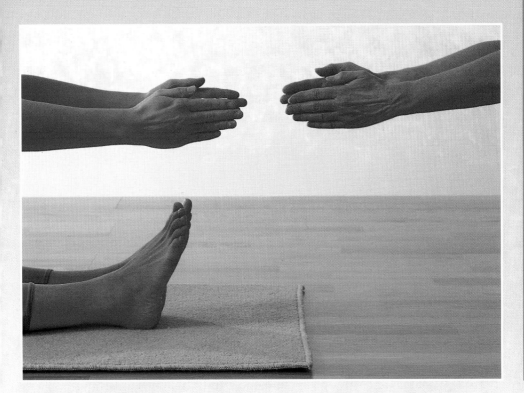

ENHANCING MENTAL AND PHYSICAL PEACE

The aim in yoga is not to imitate slavishly every technique offered but to absorb the concept and then move into your own realization. Virtually every posture can be linked with visualization to enhance both mental and physical peace and harmony.

2 Let the rhythm of your breath be the flow of your feeling of love. Each time you breathe out, allow your hands to stretch a little further forward. Soon you can feel the sensation of the fingers touching and eventually the grasp of the hands. Lose all consciousness of time. Eventually allow the vision to fade, but allow the sensation of love to remain. Finally, as you breathe in, straighten up, stretching the trunk in the air, before relaxing completely. Mind and body will feel lovingly stretched.

3 As usual, move on into the Cobra. The loving feeling can be enhanced by considering the beauties of nature. For example, bring to mind an autumn scene, full of golden tints and continue looking up at it, allowing your whole body to relax. Again, let the vision fade a little while before you come down on an out-breath and relax.

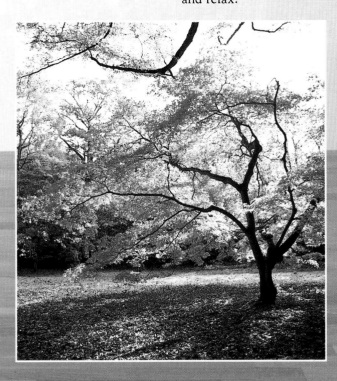

12

FITTING RELAXATION TO THE NEED

The more you progress in yoga, the more you discover that you have many means of control at your command. Asanas, visualization, meditation are all powerful tools. Relaxation, too, can be developed to enhance general well-being. It is not merely a matter of feeling good, but of actually promoting functions that are truly beneficial.

An immense range of activity is incepted as a result of messages fed to glands in the brain. Central to this activity are the hypothalamus and pituitary glands – sometimes known as the command glands of the body. Interestingly, classical yoga knowledge places a *chakra,* or energy area, at this point. It is given the name *Ajna* and is described as the command *chakra.* As signals, largely based on sensory impulses, are relayed to these glands, so they, in turn, send messages affecting virtually every aspect of our life.

Fight or Flight Response

If the message is alarming, defensive measures are brought into play. When the alarm is intense, the response is described as Fight or Flight, as a preparation for emergency action. The problem is that many unrelieved stress factors trigger aspects of this response without offering a physical form of dissipation and, as a

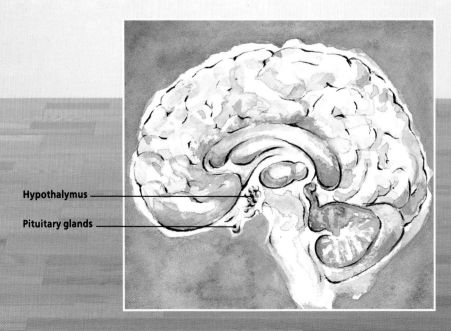

Hypothalymus

Pituitary glands

result, changes designed to be helpful become harmful instead. For example, blood sugar, released to promote energy, is not dissipated and can clog the arteries.

Relaxation Response

Other messages to the glands – those of peace and harmony – promote what is termed the Relaxation Response. Calming signals are transmitted through the body which promote balanced, healthy function.

Relaxation is an ideal way of promoting beneficial signals to the command glands. The benefits can be tremendous and far-reaching. Two important areas that have been researched so far are heart disease and high blood pressure, but many equally dangerous problems can be alleviated.

LEARNING TO RELAX

You can practise the art of relaxation at any time and any place. If you find some disturbing thought bothering you, simply sit comfortably erect, close your eyes, let your breath become slow and calm and let the disturbing thought dash itself to pieces, like a wave on the rocks. Do not expect immediate success; keep at it quietly and slowly until the right reaction occurs. Full relaxation should be used in conjunction with these briefer moments.

We now know how to lie most effectively in relaxation, keeping the physical tension to a minimum and, as a result, reducing mental tension. In relaxation we play the observer, so, while in this pose, simply bring your awareness to the head and just accept the knowledge that the brain is dealing with a never-ending supply of signals. Be aware, too, that the calmness you are introducing, linked with the peace of the breath, is affecting the response to these signals so that an alarm response becomes a relaxed and peaceful one. This is not as specific as a visualization; it is promoting a general feeling of relaxed well-being, enhanced by the effective relaxed use of the body.

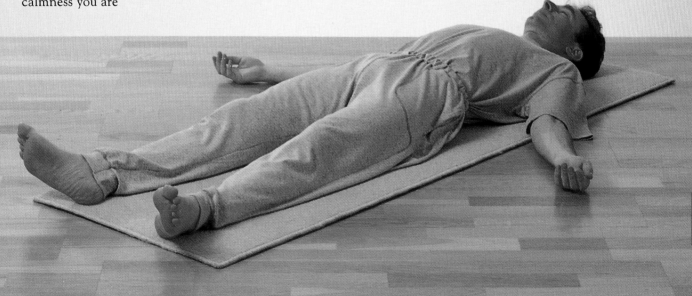

12

147

FITTING SOUND TO THE NEED

Many years ago, yogis studied the importance of sound. You know about the sound of "Om", called in Sanskrit pranava, or the primal sound, and the calming effect this sound creates. Internal sounds can also be discovered and, while there is obviously a natural explanation for them, it is amazing how beneficial they can be. A classical technique largely cuts out the external senses, helping us to link more closely with the internal.

1 Sitting comfortably erect, place a thumb firmly against each ear, blocking out external sound.

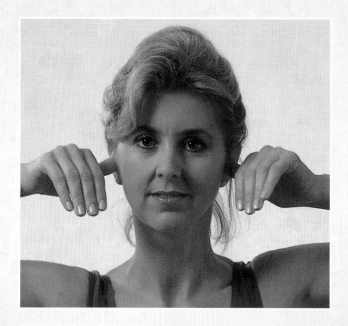

2 Now place the index fingers over the closed eyelids, cutting out sight.

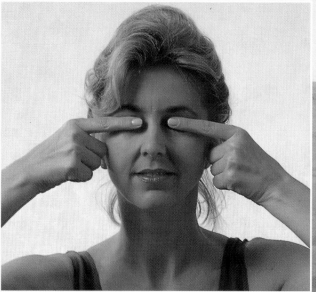

Enhancing our awareness is central to an effective life. You need to be conscious of your body, both without and within, in the same way that a managing director, in order to carry out his or her job effectively, needs to have a close knowledge of every aspect of the company's activities. All the different aspects of yoga help you to stay in touch with your body, breath, brain, mind and consciousness.

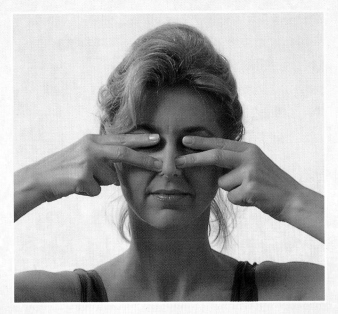

3 The second fingers rest against the nostrils, reducing the breath to a very fine and gentle process.

4 The third and fourth fingers cover the top and bottom lips, pressing them together and eliminating speech. Maintain the pressure, keeping a very gentle, fine breath. The result will be an insight into the immense internal activity that you normally never hear, with the throb of the pulse as the "beat". This is a striking reminder of the fact that within us there is an almost continuous factory-like action going on. All these activities are designed to function rhythmically. When we become ill we talk of disease – in other words, the body has moved out of ease, or its natural rhythm.

If the pressure is continued, eventually a distinguishing sound will be heard, cutting through the "factory" noises. Listening to this brings with it a sense of tranquility.

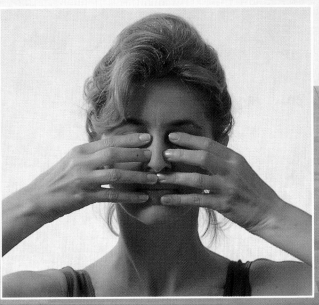

FITTING SOUND TO THE NEED

12

MOVING INTO CONTEMPLATION

Proceeding on the full path of meditation is called Raja Yoga – or the King of the Yogas. The aim is to get ever closer to the union which forms the whole basis of life. While only a few people feel called to explore this path to the full, the steps along the way are of tremendous benefit to everyone. For so much of our lives we feel that if we "get by" we are doing well. Yet always there is that nagging feeling at the back of the mind that there is something more – something wonderful to experience. Meditation begins with concentration: the ability to bring the mind to bear exclusively upon one still concept. When this becomes more and more possible (not the same as mastering it wholly), you can move on to contemplation. This can best be described as "becoming a part of".

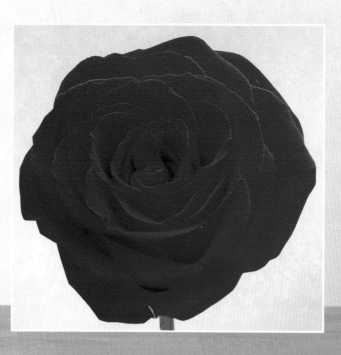

The concept of living implies action; that of being implies stillness. While we have been born human beings, we might just as well have been a tree, a bird, a flower. In developing the art of contemplation it is sensible to dwell on this thought first. This will make it easier to "be" the rose – or anything else with which you aim to become one.

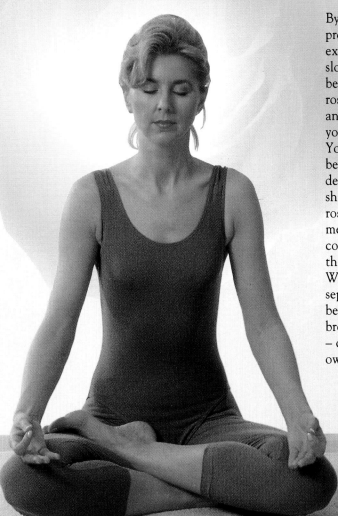

Many people find that a good object to choose for contemplation is a rose. This is one of the most loved of all flowers. The idea is to visualize a single rose, first taking in the form and the colour. Then begin to "see" the shape and linking of every individual petal. At this stage it becomes possible even to appreciate the scent of the rose. The beauty of this flower is such that you can examine it minutely with intense interest. Make sure you have settled on just one bloom – do not move away on to another flower or colour.

By continuing the process of this minute examination, you can slowly feel you are becoming a part of the rose. No longer are you an outsider observing; you have merged with it. You have taken on its beauty, you have developed its subtle shape, you are a living rose. This sense of merged identity can continue for some time – there are no limits. When you feel yourself separating once again, become aware of your breath and – very slowly – come back into your own being.

MOVING INTO CONTEMPLATION

12

"The more we learn about the universe, the more it appears to be the product of a single great thought."
**Sir James Jeans,
the eminent British physicist**

Yoga is a process by which we realize more and more fully that we are an integral part of that single great thought.
The end of this book is really just a beginning. A whole new world is in front of you waiting to be explored. Despite the claims of some scientists (by no means all), it is unlikely that we shall learn the entire truth, but there is real joy in unearthing clue after clue and finding they take us closer and closer to this concept of one-ness or union which we call yoga. I have enjoyed sharing my experiences with you through this course. Even though our paths may now diverge, the goal remains the same. I wish you joy on your journey.

Howard Kent

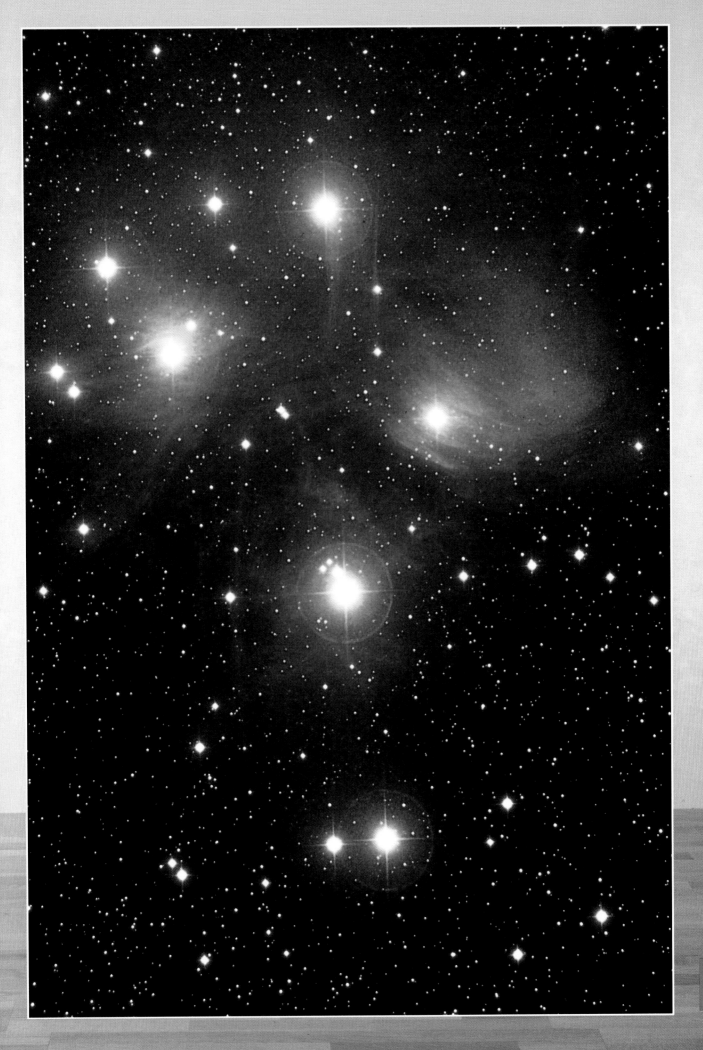

THE LANGUAGE OF YOGA

The early yoga texts were propounded in one of the world's great classical languages, Sanscrit. For a considerable period of time this was only spoken and the statements were handed down by word of mouth, being memorized and chanted. Subsequently a written form of Sanscrit appeared, which allowed the texts to be transcribed. There is absolutely no reason why the average student of yoga should seek to master the Sanscrit language, but it is useful to understand the basic terms, especially of the asanas or postures, as some teachers tend to use these exclusively.

The Postures

Posture: *Asana* (ah-sna) This means holding a position.

Bee Breath: *Brahmari*

Lotus Posture: *Padmasana* The best known of the cross-legged positions. This is one of a number of variations.

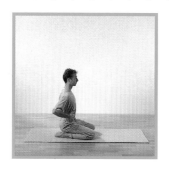

Sitting on the Heels: *Vajrasana*

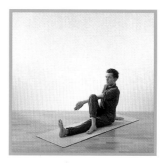

Spinal Twist: *Matsyendrasana*

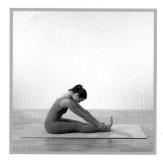

Back Body Stretch: *Paschimotanasana. Paschima* (pashima) means the West. The body is facing the East, so the West side is stretched.

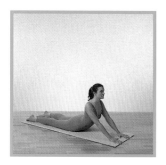

The Cobra: *Bhujangasana*

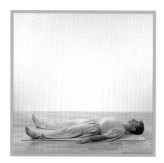

Relaxation: *Shavasana* The pose of the corpse – that is the totally limp body, after the disappearance of rigor mortis.

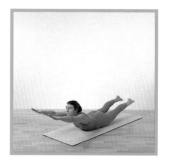

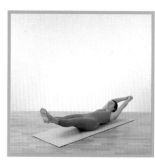

Canoe and Reverse Canoe: *Naukasana*

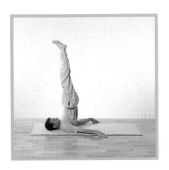

Shoulder Stand: *Sharvangasana*

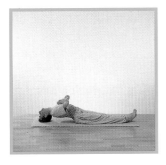

Fish: *Matsyasana*

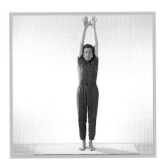

Mountain: *Parvatasana*

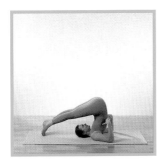

Plough: *Halasana*

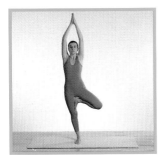

Tree: *Vrikshasana*

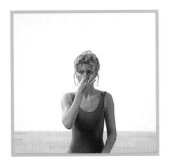

Alternate Nostril Breath: *Nadi Shuddan*
The cleansing of the subtle nervous system.

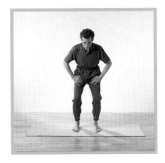

Bellows Breath: *Bastrika*
Shining Head Breath: *Kapalabhati*

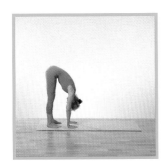

Standing Back Body Stretch: *Padhastasana*

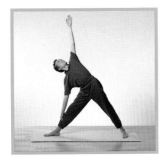

Triangle: *Trikonasana*

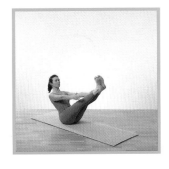

Bow: *Dhanurasana*

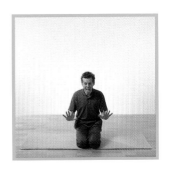

Lion: *Simbhasana*

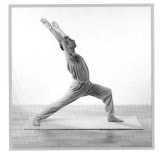

Hanuman Poses: *Vajrangasana*

(**Note:** In some cases, where there is no agreement on the correct terminology for certain postures, these have been omitted. Similarly, some of the poses shown are not classical yoga and do not have a *Sanscrit* name.)

Other useful terms
Meditation: The sequence of meditation is given as *Dharana* or concentration, *Dhyana* or contemplation and *Samadhi* or the full meditative state, super-consciousness.
Yamas: The way to relate to others – ie non-violently, truthfully, etc.
Niyamas: The way we should relate to ourselves: with equanimity, inner and outer cleanliness, devotion to the creator, etc.

Pratyahara: The ability to control the senses.
Brahmacharya: The ability to overcome lust.
Om: The primal sound of the universe – the all-connecting sound.
Yoga: One-ness, an understanding of the interlinking of everything. Also used to denote a means of reaching such an understanding, as in *Hatha Yoga*.
Chakra: A vortex of energy within the body.
Nadis: The means by which energy flows within the body.

Pronunciation
It should be remembered that in most instances the final "a" is optional: thus *asana* can also be shown as *asan*. Since *Sanscrit* has both a different alphabet and a different script, for our use it has first to be transliterated into Roman script and then translated. The result is that certain letters vary in pronunciation according to the placing of accents.

CONTINUING YOUR PRACTICE

You will have gathered that yoga is an immense subject and can be tackled in many ways. It is easy to feel somewhat threatened and confused, especially when attempts are made by some teachers to get you to believe their way is the only way.

Yoga is basically very simple: it involves letting unnecessary conditioning drop away. Little children are natural, even innocent, but adults become complex and unnatural. If you use yoga to increase the complexity, you become even more unnatural. Never forget that a technique in yoga is only an aid to reach a goal. The great classical yoga teachers point out that as you develop on the path, so techniques drop away. The aim, in other words, is not to learn more and more *asanas*, but to understand their purpose and to use them so well that you actually need them less and less.

Never forget that yoga is *self*-realization. Listen to what others – including gurus and teachers – have to say, but remember the final decisions are yours. "To thine own self be true."

Yoga is now practised virtually throughout the world. There can be relatively few places without a teacher or an organization within reach. There is, however, no single world-wide authority. Generally it will be quite easy to find what is available wherever you live but if you would like help, write to me at this address: Yoga for Health Foundation, Ickwell Bury, Biggleswade, Bedfordshire SG18 9EF, England.

The Foundation operates in many countries and can provide contacts in others. Ickwell Bury is a residential yoga centre for those studying yoga and seeking to renew their health. Enquiries always welcome.

BIBLIOGRAPHY

Very many books have been published on the subject of yoga. Unfortunately, they tend to go out of print. If this does prove to be the case it should be possible to borrow a copy through a library.

Publishers have not been listed, as these tend to vary from country to country.

Major books on Hatha Yoga include:
  Light on Yoga by B. K. S. Iyengar
  The Complete Illustrated Book of Yoga
    by Swami Vishnudevananda
  Yoga Self-Taught by André Van Lysebeth

More specialized books include:
  Yoga for the Disabled by Howard Kent
  Yoga for the Athlete by Harvey Day
  Yoga for Common Ailments
    by Drs R. Nagararhna, H. T. Nagendra
    and Robin Monro
  Easy Pregnancy with Yoga by Stella Weller
  Positive Pregnancy Fitness by Silvia Klein Olkin

A good introduction to the concept of yoga is:
  Understanding Yoga by Tom McArthur

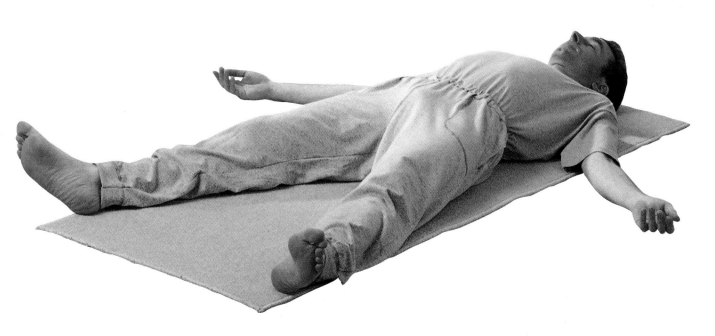

INDEX

ACKNOWLEDGMENTS

All images in this book are the copyright of Quarto Publishing
plc except for those listed below:

page 36 Life File/Jeremy Hoare; 43 Life File/Miguel Arana;
47 Life File/R Whistler; 49 Life File/Andrew Ward; 53 Life File/
R Whistler; 87 Survival Anglia/J B Davidson; 99(l) Trip/Eye
Ubiquitous; 99(b) Life File/Fergus Smith; 143 Trip/Helene
Rogers; 145 Trip/Roy Styles.

The publishers would like to thank Speedo (Europe) Ltd.